The He[a] Makeover:

How I Changed My Habits, Lost Weight, and How You Can Too

Stacy Wright

Published by

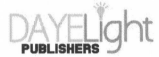

ISBN: 978-1-953759-51-1 (paperback)

The content of this book is for informational purposes only and is not intended to diagnose, treat, cure, or prevent any condition or disease. You understand that this book is not intended as a substitute for consultation with a licensed practitioner. Please consult with your own physician or healthcare specialist regarding the suggestions and recommendations made in this book. The use of this book implies your acceptance of this disclaimer.

To all those women labeled as the "fat friend," may this book bring you healing as much as it has brought me.

Acknowledgments

I would like to thank my family and friends who always supported and encouraged me to pursue my dreams no matter how big or small. No matter how much I doubted myself, you always had an encouraging word and solutions to my problems. You have always had unshakeable faith in my abilities, and for that, I am forever grateful that God placed you all in my life.

Table of Contents

Acknowledgments 5

Introduction 9

Chapter 1: Younger Me 11

Chapter 2: Food and I 17

Chapter 3: Dieting and Self Esteem 23

Chapter 4: Obesity: The Naked Truth 33

Chapter 5: Hypertension: The Naked Truth 39

Chapter 6: Time in the Valley 43

Chapter 7: Turning Pain into Purpose 51

Chapter 8: Practical Strategies about Eating Right 61

Chapter 9: Living Right 75

Chapter 10: Maintaining a Healthy Lifestyle 89

Chapter 11: COVID-19 Pandemic Weight Gain: Causes and Tips to Lose It 93

Chapter 12: Inspire U 107

Bonus Chapter: How to Start Your Own Healthy Makeover 111

Recipes 123

About the Author 127

References 129

Introduction

What exactly is a healthy makeover? When we think of makeovers, we typically think about our physical appearance. I chose the name the *Healthy Makeover* because years ago, I was desperately trying every diet to help change my size and weight. I wanted to be thin and beautiful. I wanted to be free from the fat cage that society and I had put me in. I was so fixated on my physical appearance I never once thought about my insides—my emotional and mental well-being and how genetics and my relationship with food were affecting my health.

Does this sound like you? Tried diet after diet and in a matter of time you gained back all the weight and more? Me too. After dieting for only two days, you give up and immediately started bingeing on comfort foods to recover from the starvation? Yes, I did that too. Are you ready to come off the diet Ferris Wheel and focus on changing your habits that you can maintain longer term? If your answer is yes, then this book is for you.

The Healthy Makeover is a detailed story of how I battled obesity from my childhood to late twenties and its impact on my self-esteem. This is an overview of my past dieting habits driven by my unhealthy desire to be thin. Additionally you will also get detailed insight on how I dealt with the pain of ending a relationship, anxiety and hypertension while living in Japan. With all these experiences compounded, they forced me to take a serious look at my health. Consequently, I employed strategies that helped me to get back in control and finally lose the weight while simultaneously maintaining my lifestyle for so many years, even during the midst of a pandemic. As a bonus, I provided you with some easy tips and delicious recipes to help you to begin your own healthy makeover journey!

This book is not another diet or quick tool to show you how to lose weight but a guide on how you can start assessing your own habits and helping you to replace any unhealthy ones with healthier habits you can maintain for the long haul.

Writing this book has been so cathartic; it has helped to heal and release emotions I thought I overcame. My hope is that this book will encourage, inspire, and motivate you to take your health seriously no matter your age or health status. We all have things that we need to improve on no matter how small. This book has been in the making for a long time, and I am deeply honored you picked this book, my book to read.

Happy reading and happy healthy makeover!

Chapter 1

Younger Me

"Look at fatty jump!" a man shouted. He was watching from the sidelines as I successfully jumped over the horizontal rope during the high jump event at the annual Sports Day at my preparatory school. As I type these words, I can clearly remember everything about that moment. Families and friends all gathered cheering and applauding after each successful jump, as the rope got higher and higher. While the height of the rope eludes me, I surely recall it was too tall for the average eight-year-old to jump over. I was confident in my abilities; after all, we practiced thoroughly for this very day. However, those four words "look at fatty jump" managed to silence the crowd and burrowed itself within the deep crevices of my mind. They served as a constant reminder that my talents and skills will always be overshadowed by my weight.

I do not know if it was that particular event that triggered the self-consciousness of my body and weight, but for years to come, my weight would be a persistent topic that would pervade every area of my life. No one chooses to be overweight; as stated by Harvard Health, your weight is contingent on calorie consumption and how many calories your body stores and burns (Health, 2019), with each of these factors being influenced by genetics and the environment.

The interrelation between all these factors starts from conception and continues throughout life (Health, 2019).

Have you ever watched the television show on the TLC Channel called "*My 600 lb. Life?*" It is a documentary that follows persons who are morbidly obese and their journey to losing weight. A lot of us tend to judge people for their weight and attribute it to the simple fact of overeating. However, if you watch shows like the aforementioned, it shows that it is much deeper than "eating too much." Someone's weight and size are only the outer layer of a weight issue. Like an onion, you must peel back the layers to get to the center or root cause of obesity. So, here's my story.

In retrospect, my childhood, I had what many would say was a privileged upbringing. I was born in the eighties in St. Andrew, Jamaica, the first child for my mother but the third for my father. As the new baby, I was adored and spoilt with any and everything. I was raised in an upper-middle-class home. Therefore, I had the typical lifestyle of attending the best schools in Jamaica and receiving a well-rounded education. I was exposed to ballet, swimming, and tennis lessons with access to private tutors.

Outside of school, I was just as busy. I was a member of my school's swim team as well as the Tornadoes Swim Club, one of the top competitive swimming clubs in Kingston. We had swim practice after school a few times weekly and early mornings on Saturdays. We had additional practices whenever I had to participate in swimming competitions locally and even abroad. I had the ideal life. However, despite my level of athleticism at such a young age, society was only and always fixated on my physical image and weight.

Even though I was involved and exposed in various activities, I was a shy and introverted child. I was described by many as quiet, well-mannered, calm, and someone who only "speaks when spoken to." While at home, I showed a slightly different side. I was more outspoken, goofy, and free-spirited. According to a Japanese proverb, we have three faces. The first face is the one you show the world; the second, you show to your family and close friends; and the third face, you never show anyone. It is this face that represents the truest reflection of who you are. Do you agree? I think for me, and possibly many of us, I feel comfortable to be my most authentic self around those who accept me and are less likely to judge and criticize. Looking back, I did not realize it then, but within the middle and upper-class society of Jamaica, being fat was frowned upon.

Weight in Jamaican Society

In today's society, we are seeing this global trend of body positivity—women embracing and accepting their own bodies while concurrently challenging society's views on this issue. The aim of this body positivity movement is to help people understand how popular media messages contribute to the relationship that people have with their bodies. Growing up, I never had these types of discussions or messages. Like most young girls, I struggled with my body image and felt I had more insecurities for being overweight, particularly in middle-class Jamaica.

In every country, there are certain cultural norms and societal nuances that are unspoken yet understood. As a light-skinned black woman, issues of colorism and privilege were not obvious to me as a young girl as a majority of my friends and those within my social circle looked like me. Despite the opportunities being fair-skinned seemly afforded me, according to some, I felt it did not matter because in my own circle I was judged and overlooked because of my weight.

I was always the fat friend among my group of friends from prep school straight through to college. Therefore, I was invisible. Particularly among the popular girls and boys that I desperately wanted to like me. As I mentioned earlier, I was involved in several extracurricular activities, particularly swimming, and I associated with the popular kids, yet I never fit in. I was shy, even intimidated as I saw that I never "looked" like them. I was good at swimming and won numerous medals but the subconscious gnawing of not being good enough because of my weight caused me so much anxiety that it played a major role in my decision to give up competitive swimming. I got tired of the rigorous routine, late evenings, and early weekend mornings. I always had an upset stomach on competition days; it was too much. Despite the lectures and pleading from my swim coaches and mother, after a few years, I was done. I wanted to do something else that made me happy. By the time I got to high school, I had become more interested in activities that developed my artistic, social, and leadership skills, as physical appearance was not the center of attention.

My insecurities only got worse during my teenage years. Luckily, school uniforms are a requirement in Jamaica, so I never had to worry about what to wear to school. However, on those special occasions like Jeans Day or Fun Day when we were allowed to wear our own clothes, I struggled so much. My room would look like a hurricane had passed through it as I could never find anything to wear. My clothes weren't hip or trendy, and if it was in style, I definitely did not look like my friends. I would cry, fearing the worst. Negative thoughts I believed and heard about myself would come rushing back, "Look at fatty jump!" This cycle of self-hate continued every single time I had to go to a social event.

I am so happy to see how much times have changed and improved as more stores and brands have become inclusive. Finding clothes was difficult in the '90s because everything for a plus-sized child/teenager was nearly impossible to find. The options were not only limited but outdated. The majority of my clothes were made by a dressmaker or were adult-sized. The sheer difficulty I had to deal with in order to pick out clothes and find something that actually fit made me awkward and uncomfortable in social settings. Instead of focusing on my friends and having a great time, I was fixated on what everyone thought of me and wishing I would look like someone else.

Naturally, low self-esteem spilled over into other areas of my life, and my self-consciousness about my appearance prevented me from wanting to do things. In kindergarten and high school, I aspired to be a cheerleader. I loved the idea of wearing the costumes and learning the dancing routines; it looked so fun and liberating. I refrained from telling anyone of my interest because they would reiterate the exact thoughts I kept reminding myself, "Fat people can't be cheerleaders." Furthermore, I visualized people laughing and teasing me. Mortified, I chose activities that would make me less noticeable and admired from afar those cheerleaders who beamed with confidence.

As I finished my last couple of years in high school, I branched out more as I was comfortable with my friends and the school environment. I became more involved in various activities but made sure it was not too much outside of my comfort zone. I did things that made people laugh and was known as the sweet yet goofy girl. During skits and plays, I gravitated towards roles that were typical for a fat person or were guaranteed to make others laugh. I ensured that whatever I did, I would make others laugh with me and not at me.

When it came time to decide what I wanted to do after high school, I knew right away I wanted to go to college far, far away from Jamaica. This would be the perfect time to start over and be someone else—be who I was supposed to be.

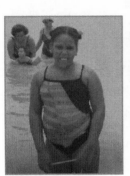
At the beach

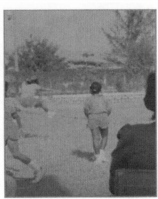
Kindergarten Sports Day

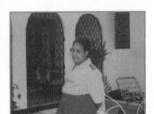
High School

Chapter 1 Quotes:

- ❖ "Happiness isn't size specific." —Ana Guest-Jelley
- ❖ "There is no weight limit on beauty." —Anonymous
- ❖ "My body is a part of who I am, but it isn't everything." —Molly Ho
- ❖ "Build a strong mindset. The body will follow." — Anonymous

Chapter 2

Food and I

When I made the decision to attend Ithaca College in New York to pursue my undergraduate degree, I was overjoyed. I would be far away in a place where no one knew me. This was the perfect opportunity to reinvent myself. The day I left Jamaica, I never cried nor looked back. I barely hugged my family goodbye. This was the time I could be myself.

The first week of school was filled with orientation sessions about college life. One of the topics of discussion was the dreaded "Freshmen 15." For those of you who do not know, during the first year of college in the US, an estimated 50% of students will gain up to fifteen pounds as a result of poor dietary choices, limited knowledge of nutritional requirements combined with partying and alcohol consumption (Deliens, 2014). That was not good news for someone who was already overweight. When I started school, I was approximately two hundred pounds and wearing a US size 18/20 in clothes.

Surprisingly, I actually lost weight in my first semester. I do not remember how much weight I lost, but I went from a size 18/20 down to a size 14/12 while everyone else around me gained weight. I ate the same foods everyone else ate. I basked in the comfort of foods that I knew, pizza and ice cream late at nights, and alcohol almost every weekend. So, what did I do differently? It may have been due to the change in the environment. Ithaca is located in Central New York, close to the border of Canada and roughly four to five hours away from New York City. The campus is situated on the South Hill and within walking distance between the classrooms and dorms. To get off campus was just as convenient as certain shops and nightlife activities were just as accessible on foot or by bus. Coming from Jamaica where we drove everywhere, to having to walk and utilize public transportation to go everywhere was new to me and was the main contributor to losing weight.

Unfortunately, my amazing weight loss did not last too long. By the end of my four years, I had gained back most of my weight. I tried very hard throughout the time to maintain it. I started going to the gym and focused on what I was eating. I began eating salads for lunch and dinner, incorporated fresh fruits for breakfast, and reduced my carb and sugar intake as much as possible. My eating habits in college were definitely unhealthy but a significant improvement in comparison to my dietary habits growing up.

My poor eating habits were multi-factorial, one reason being, I was a very picky eater. Looking at me, the automatic assumption is that I loved any and all foods and in large quantities. However, that was not true. In comparison to my family members, I was definitely the outlier. My family shared stories of me being fed chicken and refusing to swallow it because I could not tolerate the texture. Apparently, it would take me hours to break it down. My mother tried feeding me an assortment of foods; I refused a lot of it. I was more tolerant of junk and processed foods, possibly for psychological reasons. In a 2015 article titled, *"Why kids want to eat processed foods (& how to change that),"* it explains that the human brain has a neural structure called "the reward system" (Harding, 2017). This exists to reward us with a lot of feel-good chemicals like dopamine when we do something that improves our chance of survival-like eating (Harding, 2017). "Therefore, children's brains are biologically hardwired to seek out foods that stimulate the reward system" (Harding, 2017). Research also indicates that as kids continue learning and developing, their taste buds should improve and stabilize to appreciate more foods (Jacewicz, 2017). This is not the moment where I can happily state by the time I reached age ten I finally began my love affair with chicken. I still hated it. I had no desire for chicken or other meats and was just as finicky with other wholesome food groups. My diet for roughly twenty years was very selective and consisted only of foods I enjoyed, which was limited to processed and junk foods. I ate vegetables occasionally, and by occasionally, I mean the one or two lettuce leaves in the Burger King Whopper or as the obligatory side option for Sunday dinner. My finicky eating habits were not that much different from other kids, but my aversion to so many commonly eaten foods was utterly mind-boggling to my family members.

Comparatively speaking, the dietary practices of my mother were no different between my younger brother and me. However, his eating habits were not persnickety. My brother was skinner than I ever was growing up, and we were both just as physically active. What went wrong with me, I wondered? Why was I more predisposed to being overweight?

Why Did I Become Fat?

I was born weighing roughly six pounds, an average-sized healthy baby. Being the first child for my mother, adoration did not stop at clothes and toys but it continued with food. I recall being told that my aunt, my mother's sister, would feed me even when I was not hungry. If my mother wanted to give me water, my aunt gave me juice instead. My aunt was more likely to shower me with sweet treats, yet she was more rigid when it came to food waste. Every time I visited her, I had to finish everything on the plate. Sadly, the amount of food on the plate was way more than I could finish at times. I totally understand wasting food is not good given how expensive it is, but overfeeding a child is not good either.

I was picky about what I ate, and the only meat I enjoyed was ground beef. I loved beef patties (a savory pastry filled with ground beef, similar to empanadas) and other processed foods like vienna sausages and bologna. If I was not eating a patty, I would eat baked macaroni and cheese. While everyone else had a well-balanced plate, mine was filled with carbohydrates. I would eat macaroni and cheese with a small serving of rice only and maybe two leaves of lettuce for balance. This was what my meals looked like for years. Ice cream was another guilty pleasure that brought satisfaction to my soul. I found comfort and joy in every single scoop. Unfortunately, my adoration for sweets did not stop at ice cream. This also included chocolate, cakes, and sweet teas. I have fond memories of my grandmother and I chatting and making black tea with condensed milk. The tea would be black and turned white because of the amount of condensed milk we added. It was far from healthy, but it tasted amazing and represented fond memories that made me develop an unhealthy relationship with food.

Like many kids, I detested a lot of fruits and vegetables and limited them to select items like bananas and lettuce. Unfortunately, as I got older, my desire to step out and try new foods was a struggle. I even refused to try ordinary everyday foods. In hindsight, my strong resistance and possible disdain for certain foods could only be explained by a psychological barrier that would trigger a physical reaction of my throat closing, thereby preventing me from swallowing, which explained my inability for years to take pills. I think this was why I never opened myself to trying new things. Therefore, I stayed within the safe boundaries of what was familiar.

My parents were naturally concerned about my eating habits. Compared to my brother, who ate any and everything, I was a cause for concern, yet I was healthy according to my annual wellness check-ups. Fortunately, in college, I was exposed to a wider variety of foods and was at a phase and stage where I was ready to become the person I was supposed to be. Throughout the four years, I stuck to foods that I was accustomed to but slowly opened my palate to other foods and gained a basic understanding about nutrition.

As a young woman in the working world and especially living in New York, I tried a variety of culinary dishes. However, when I cooked for myself, I resorted to what I knew and could afford. Now that I was solely responsible for my nutritional health needs, it became apparent that my weight was still out of control, and I always relied on dieting to fix the problem.

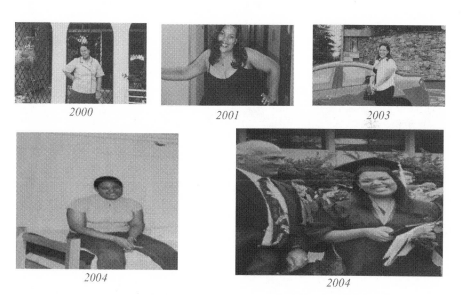

2000

2001

2003

2004

2004

Chapter 2 Quotes:

- ❖ "Food is fabulous, and having a good relationship with it will make you healthy and happy." —Denise Austin
- ❖ "Free yourself from the diet mentality to create space for a healthy relationship with food and your body." —Jennifer Bolus
- ❖ "Making peace with food requires that you transition from a place of fear to a place of love." —Anta Johnston
- ❖ "We're taught ridiculous strategies for fending off cravings, everything from eating carrot sticks to tapping on our forehead. But we're never taught skills to competently eat all foods." —The Joy of Eating

Chapter 3

Dieting and Self Esteem

As mentioned previously, research studies have substantiated that a child's health, specifically dietary and physical behaviors, are influenced by parenting and the home environment (Duke Medicine, 2013) (Pyper, 2016). My mother, for as long as I can remember, was and still is a dedicated gym member. As a little girl, I would sit on the sidelines and watch her impressively jump, kick and side shuffle during aerobic classes. My mother took pride in her appearance, and I always admired the way she carried herself with style, grace, and sophistication that still stands to this day. I wanted to be like her.

Her ability to maintain her size 8/10 frame was not only because of her dedication to exercise but also because of her eating habits. She always had a balanced meal and indulged in the occasional sweet treats. I remember her stories of growing up, despising the slightest hint of anyone calling her "chubby" or 'fat," which instantly propelled her to go into diet mode. Like most of us, she was another victim of diet culture that I eventually adopted to deal with unwanted weight gain. I was hooked when I saw that I could lose as much as ten pounds in just seven days. One new customer boarding the toxic diet express train. Destination, obsession, and self-hate!

The first diet ever tried was the cabbage soup diet, AKA "Wonder Soup" or "Military Diet." This diet guaranteed I would lose weight fast. I immediately began visualizing myself as a completely new person. I would start early summer, naively imagining myself fifty pounds lighter in a matter of weeks. By the time I would return to school, all my friends would be praising me, and the boys I had crushes on would finally like me back. I put all my hopes and dreams of being skinny in a big pot of fowl-smelling soup. I never knew that cabbage could smell so bad cooked (no offense to cabbage lovers). But, it really did not smell good even combined with the other vegetables and seasonings. Meals were limited to specific fruits and vegetables with unlimited servings of this miracle soup. I hated every second of it. Day one could not end quickly enough; imagine six more days of this. I forced myself not to think about it and instead visualized being slim and wearing the hottest of outfits and having all the boys salivating over me. The only person left drooling was me, as I dug into a bowl of ice cream by the end of day three. I gave up because I was so hungry and detested the soup. If this is what it takes to look good, this soup was not worth it.

Foolishly, I tried this diet on several occasions and possibly lasted a full week only once. By the eighth day, I went right back to my old eating habits because I was relieved to be eating real food again. It was like a reward for the punishment I placed myself in while completely forgetting the reason I was starving myself in the first place.

This unhealthy cycle of dieting always came after moments of feeling disgusted and ashamed at how I looked. I started and stopped the diets that were just too difficult within three days; I constantly felt deprived. When I failed, I felt as if being skinny was just not in my destiny, and I would forever be labeled as, "that fat girl" or as the "fat friend." I vicariously lived my life through television shows and even novels. I felt drawn to storylines of girls who were labeled as plump or overweight and, magically, over that one summer before attending high school, became skinny and instantly popular. In reality, over the summers, I gained weight.

The most consistent program I have tried was *Herbalife*. *Herbalife* is an extremely successful and world-renowned business that is used and distributed in Jamaica. They offer a variety of nutritional programs that can be created based on the goals you have in mind, such as weight gain, maintenance, and weight loss. The weight-loss program consists of a protein shake that I would drink twice per day and then one fully balanced meal. Additionally, I would need to take a couple of supplements and teas for cellular activation and energy promotion. I found this program to be less restrictive and manageable. I loved the shakes because they were delicious and tasted like milkshakes. The only downfall was, I hated the tablets. The required dosage was 3 to 4 pills per day, which was unacceptable in my book.

The products were always at my disposal because my mom was a customer and distributor. However, I was not a consistent user mainly because of the size of the pills and the fact that they were necessary components for weight loss. My mom and my aunt even resorted to adding the pills to the shakes so I would not have to worry about taking them. Bad idea. It made the shakes look unappealing. To a young pre-teen, it was like vegetables in liquid form and medicine in one. Upon reflection, I honestly think I could have been successful with this program, but I was still in that phase where I was so particular about what I ate that anything outside of what I knew was just unacceptable. However, as an adult, I was satisfied with drinking the protein shakes mainly out of convenience during working hours when I needed something light and simple. I eventually stopped using the products as I found other alternatives.

I became aware of new diet crazes through the media and, of course, friends and family. I tried diets where you drink natural fruit juices only, teas with laxatives for bloating and weight loss. I never tried diet pills or injections containing chemicals or hormones to aid in weight loss, probably because of my aversion to pills. Personally, that was not something I felt was safe for my body, and I was aware of the potential side effects. I was curious but never comfortable enough to try it.

With every diet, I was always hungry, angry, and secretly wanting to strangle people as I watched them enjoy foods I wanted to be eating. Each diet I tried, I failed by the third day because of how restrictive they were. I yearned for something that would make me lose weight and be satiated at the same time.

The most successful diet I tried was the South Beach Diet. The South Beach Diet was created in 2003. In the spring of 2005, I decided to try this diet after feeling fed up with having gained weight yet again. I had lost weight so effortlessly in my first year of college. Now, I was "wiser but fatter" (Preidt, 2016). Weight gain in college is to be expected, according to a 2016 study conducted by the Journal of Nutrition Education and Behavior. The study claims that students can gain on average ten pounds over the four years (Preidt, 2016).

I was now a college graduate, paying my own bills and earning a decent salary in New York City. I was determined this time to stick with this program as it seemed manageable, not as restrictive, and offered a wide variety of recipes that promoted weight loss. It was the most rewarding as I could continue to enjoy foods such as cheese and yogurt. The South Beach Diet has three phases. The first phase, which lasts for two weeks, requires that you eliminate all carbohydrates and sugar and eat foods high in protein and fat along with limited fruits and vegetables. The second phase, which was the third week, slowly incorporated healthy carbs, and the last phase, the maintenance phase, is where you enjoy all foods in moderation. I maintained the diet for roughly three months following the first phase only and lost roughly thirty pounds without regular exercise. I did not want to try the other phases until I felt I had lost more weight. I was consistent and developed an eating routine that worked. However, that routine would be disrupted by an unforeseen change in my life's plan. By the summer of 2005, I begrudgingly left NYC and moved back to Jamaica. I was so bitter about being back home and worried about what I would be doing next; I lost interest in losing weight. Without realizing it, my old habits crept in, and all the weight and more came right back, again.

Despite the setback, for the very first time I was so successful on a diet. Even though I lost weight before, this was the first diet that I successfully maintained. I made several attempts to restart the South Beach Diet over the next few years, but I could not go beyond a week. The many times after felt extremely difficult as my desire to lose weight was not as strong as my love for food. Unfortunately, every time I was unable to lose the weight, the negative thoughts came knocking on the door of my mind. I felt ugly, unwanted, unloved, and like a failure.

How was I able to lose weight in the past and not now? Was my willpower not strong enough? Did I lack motivation? Were my reasons for losing weight not strong motivators? When it comes to weight management, I believe it is a very complex subject matter that goes beyond "eating too much." For some people, they might have weight problems because of metabolic or hormonal conditions that require medical assistance. In my case, I believe I had unhealthy eating habits, limited knowledge and awareness, coupled with poor self-esteem.

People lose weight all the time. I lost weight before; what was different this time? Was it my willpower? What is willpower? According to Kelly McGonigal, PhD, a health psychologist at Stanford University who specializes in mind-body connection, willpower is a "mind-body response" and "a reaction to an internal conflict" (Steakley, 2011). We all have willpower, but according to McGonigal, when we are under stress, it is more difficult to have willpower (Steakley, 2011). Stress and willpower are conflicting within our bodies; stress "encourages you to focus on immediate, short-term goals and outcomes, but self-control requires keeping the big picture in mind" (Steakley, 2011). Thinking about this and every time I dieted throughout my life, I had to ask myself if I was under some form of stress.

Can dieting be considered a form of stress? A number of doctors think so, including Dr. Pamela Peeke. Dr. Peeke's article, *"Dieting is Stressful: Ditch the Diet Mentality,"* points out the various things that make us anxious when we go on a diet. Mentioned were breaking out into hives, looking at a bathroom scale, feeling hopeless about your clothing size, counting calories, worrying about resisting certain foods when out at social events, and having feelings of guilt and shame after looking for food late at night (Peeke, 2010). As a result, stress increases cortisol (stress hormone) which prevents you from losing weight (Peeke, 2010).

Combining the theories by both McGonigal and Peeke, I would say I was fixated on my unrealistic goal of losing weight instantaneously; I was doing more harm than good. As a teenager, my motive for losing weight was purely superficial and routed in low self-esteem. I wanted to lose weight because I wanted to wear clothes that were in style; I wanted to look like the girls I went to school with, and I wanted to be considered attractive and noticed by boys. I was obsessed with these reasons each time I started a diet, but I became frustrated when I did not magically appear to be fifty pounds lighter by the second or third day of starving myself. I became frustrated when the scale would not move and when my jeans pants still squeezed the life out of me. I was emotionally exhausted after fifteen minutes crying sessions, and I still hated the reflection staring at me in the mirror. Therefore, I gave up! Losing weight was too difficult.

Being overweight dictated who I was supposed to be, how people saw me, and how people interacted with me. I wanted to be liked. Ironically, I was liked by a lot of persons and labeled as the sweet, kind, nice, quiet, long-haired girl. These were all great qualities, but I felt invisible. I felt like no one truly saw me. Being overweight placed me in the proverbial box that I willingly accepted.

In kindergarten, we had a school play about Winnie the Pooh; the entire class had to participate no matter the role. My classmates and I all naturally thought I would play the character of Pooh, especially since I looked the part. We were all wrong; I played a honeybee. However, in my senior year at high school, I played the part of our school principal, who was heavyset and wore glasses like me. I did not necessarily want to act that part, so I do not know why it was given to me. Maybe it was because I had the same physical characteristics as the principal. No one said anything, but I made that assumption and it hurt. In my eyes, I could only identify with qualities I hated about myself. Now I am proud to have played the role of a woman who was a strong leader. Navigating my role within my friend's groups was not without issues as well.

I had genuine friendships growing up that helped shape and mold me into the person I am today. In spite of this, I could never shake my role as the token "fat friend." As an undergrad, I was lucky enough to have friends who came from Jamaica, which made the transition so much easier. We all bonded over this major milestone attending this predominantly white college. Out of all six of us, I was the only one who was overweight. My friends were attractive girls who appeared exotic to everyone. They were slim built, beautiful, smart, outgoing, and exuded confidence. Yet, they had insecurities just like me. I never felt comforted within myself that they struggled with issues with their bodies; instead, I was angry whenever they complained about being fat. "If they think they're fat now, what would they say if they were my size?" I wondered. They were not fat, not even close. They never struggled with finding clothes or hated taking pictures or ensuring that their bodies were hidden as much as possible in pictures. I was so self-conscious about my body it affected people's perception of me.

I was most often overlooked and merely tolerated. No one said this verbally, but the body language and treatment said something different. Boys I had crushes on never reciprocated. They had crushes on my friends instead. I was never a threat or seen as competition. I was unmemorable and usually the source of teasing. For my four years I was given horrible nicknames that was the source of comedic relief but secretly hurt me to my core. In Jamaica, we tend to give nicknames to persons based on their most unique or pronounced feature and characteristic. For example, a guy who has a speech impediment like a stammer would be called "stamma" or a guy with one arm would be called "One-y." This type of behavior has been so normalized in Jamaican culture that we have become so blind to how damaging and toxic it can be to a person's self-esteem. Among my friends, no one else was given nicknames that referred to their size and weight except me. No matter how I shared my simple requests, my pleas to stop were ignored and laughed off. Another blow to my self-esteem, I felt unheard and disrespected.

My low self-esteem infested so many areas of my life. For many years, I never thought I was smart enough, pretty enough, or good enough for anything. I focused so much on what was wrong instead of what was right. Even if I was complimented in an area of my life, I would not believe it. When I had my first boyfriend at nineteen years old, I was surprised that any guy would like me. I was accustomed to being overlooked for so many years. I found it unbelievable that I could be liked beyond the physical appearance. Upon reflection, in a number of my relationships, including that first boyfriend, I recognize that I did not truly like any of those guys. My true, authentic self did not want them or even thought they were good enough, but my insecurities allowed me to settle and reassured me that "they're not so bad."

It was evident that from this approach my priority was only about being validated and accepted by society, when in fact the focus should have been to learn and understand the root causes of obesity and underlining factors in my life.

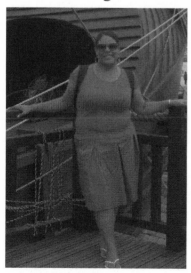 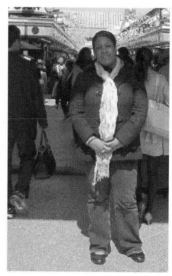

Chapter 3 Quotes:

- ❖ "It's unbelievable how enough you are." —Anonymous
- ❖ "I must undertake to love myself and to respect myself as though my very life depends upon self-love and self-respect." —Maya Angelou
- ❖ "I hate dieting. Let's just say that." —Shay Mitchell

Chapter 4

Obesity: The Naked Truth

Typically, I have been described as fat or overweight but in actuality, I was obese. Is there a difference? Technically, yes. According to the Center for Disease Control (CDC), if a person's weight is higher than the standard weight for their height, they are classified as overweight or obese. You can identify your weight classification by calculating your Body Mass Index (BMI). Your BMI is your weight, "in kilograms divided by the square of height in meters" (CDC, 2021). Doing the calculation manually is way too much, so to make life easier, there are numerous apps or online tools that can be used to calculate it for you.

The recommended or normal BMI range is 18.5 to 25 (CDC, 2021). A person whose BMI is greater than 25 but less than 30 is considered overweight, and anyone with a BMI over 30 and higher is considered obese (CDC, 2021). Furthermore, obesity has been subdivided into three categories or classes: Class 1, BMI 30 to 35; Class 2, BMI 35 to 40; and Class 3, BMI 40 or higher (CDC, 2021). When I was at my heaviest, I would have been classified as severely obese. At my heaviest, I was around 260 pounds with a BMI of 43.

The causes of obesity and being overweight are multifaceted. The main culprits are consuming too many foods in excessive quantities that are high in fat and sugars, combined with living a sedentary lifestyle. Other causalities are beyond overeating and may be attributed to genetics and underlying medical conditions. Obesity is a huge problem globally as the rates have tripled since 1975, according to the World Health Organization (WHO). The WHO reported that in 2016, over 1.9 billion adults 18 years and over were overweight, and of this figure, 650 million were obese (WHO, 2021). Obesity is not just a problem for adults but for children as well, and the numbers are just as staggering. In 2016, 41 million children under the age of five were classified as overweight or obese, while more than 340 million children and adolescents between the ages of 5 and 19 were overweight and obese (WHO, 2021).

In my native island of Jamaica and the wider Caribbean region, the statistics are equally egregious. According to a report by the "*Panorama of Food and Nutrition Security,*" in Latin America and the Caribbean, an estimated 140 million persons or 23 percent of persons are obese with the highest rates being found within countries like Barbados (36%), Trinidad and Tobago and Antigua and Barbuda (31%). Additionally, the report noted that obesity affects women more than men (10 % more) (Jamaica Observer, 2017).

The statistics in Jamaica are just as alarming. Based on the results from the *Jamaica Health and Lifestyle* survey in 2018, more than half (54%) of Jamaicans are overweight and pre-obese, with obesity affecting women on a larger scale (Jamaica Observer, 2017). What does this mean, and why am I telling you this? The reason behind the global concern about the obesity epidemic is the numerous health conditions associated with obesity, such as diabetes, high blood pressure, high cholesterol, heart disease, cancers, and sleep disorders. Many of these diseases are common in adults but are actually being diagnosed in children as well. In a 2015 study done by Jane Chiang, 1 in 3 persons less than 18 years of age will be newly diagnosed with type 2 diabetes (Chiang, 2015). Furthermore, the consequences of obesity in young children and adolescents also include early puberty, increased incidences of metabolic syndrome, and obesity in adulthood (Biro, 2010).

What seems to have a lot less public health outcry are the mental repercussions of being obese. Obese children are more likely to suffer from a psychiatric disorder, depression, behavioral problems, and social marginalization and victimization from bullying (BeLue, 2009). In a study completed by Rhonda BeLue et al titled, *"Mental Health Problems and Overweight in a Nationally Representative Sample of Adolescents: Effects of Race and Ethnicity,"* girls showed greater concern about their weight and experienced depressive symptoms when compared to those children who were overweight or obese and not concerned about their weight (BeLue, 2009). Not to say that boys and men do not have struggles with body image, but girls and women are constantly being bombarded with images and messages to look a certain way (BeLue, 2009).

Furthermore, women tend to engage in something called "Fat Talk" (Whitbourne, 2013). Societal norms exert pressure on women to feel bad about their bodies and discuss those bad feelings. The more women talk about these feelings, the higher the likelihood that fat-talking will infiltrate their self-esteem (Whitbourne, 2013). That societal pressure is further exacerbated through social media, as people can now sit behind a screen and anonymously say hateful things to women without any ramifications. Fortunately, you can delete and block trolls and send them packing forever in cyberspace, never having to deal with them again. Thank you, next. However, what do you do in real life with people you live, interact and work with on a daily basis? The belief of being seen as *less than* and not *good enough* is rampant within the Jamaican culture as well as other Black and Afro-Caribbean communities. These are beliefs and attitudes that have been perpetuated from slavery. I have had countless discussions with friends and heard testimonies from other women of relatives, friends, coworkers, and even strangers making comments or statements that would send us all spiraling down an emotional black hole. I remember specifically while on vacation visiting a new city in Japan with one of my friends. We made arrangements to stay with her friend, who I was meeting for the first time. Within 48 hours of the vacation, we were having a casual conversation about my peculiar eating habits, and I mentioned my disgust for certain foods but love or preference for vegetables. The person murmured, "then why yuh so fat then?" Although she did not intend for me to hear it, unfortunately, I did. Sadly, I felt uncomfortable for the rest of my trip. These distasteful comments can even be expected from medical professionals who are supposed to be trained to guide and help their patients. Typically, when patients visit their doctors, they expect some level of support and tact in their approach. Instead, many have planted a seed of self-hate or further aided self-destructive behaviors. For example, during my teenage years, I was a patient of a well-renowned dermatologist in Jamaica. On one particular visit, this doctor at the end of the appointment reminded me that I "need to lose some weight, girlfriend." As a teenager who had been overweight for years, tried and failed several diets, and struggling with my body image, hearing that I needed to lose weight was unnecessary and actually prolonged my unhealthy eating and lifestyle habits.

Telling someone they need to lose weight is like telling a blind person they are blind. I felt so horrible as it reminded me of my inability to lose weight, despite my best efforts. I never saw that doctor again; in fact, I stayed far away from all doctors because I didn't want to feel that level of shame again.

I knew I was overweight, and I wanted to lose the weight. It was just so difficult for me. I was the only one out of my siblings who really suffered the most with weight for many years. Was it genetic? No. If I go through my genealogy, my grandparents, in their younger days, were slim; even my parents and their siblings. My mother's sister is the only one who, for as long as I have known her, has always been overweight. Interestingly enough, despite my family members' apparent slim statures, lifestyle diseases such as heart disease, hypertension, and diabetes plagued my family. I was overly concerned with weight but not concerned enough about its impact on my health. I always knew about conditions like high blood pressure and diabetes and assumed they were a part of the aging process, but I could not comprehend the dangers of these conditions.

Chapter 4 Quotes:

❖ "Obesity affects every aspect of people's lives, from health to relationships." Jane Velez-Mitchell
❖ "When you talk about obesity, there's so many things that can cause that. It can be a medical thing or down to the individual. There's a lot of other things involved than eating a mars bar." - Peter Shilton

Chapter 5

Hypertension: The Naked Truth

always assumed that hypertension was a disease for the elderly. Being diagnosed with high blood pressure at twenty-seven years of age was a huge wake-up call. It was the slap in the face I needed to show me that my current way of doing things was not working. At first, I summed it up to genetics and trivialized it. Everyone has high blood pressure, so what's the big deal? Before I get to that, let's first understand, what is blood pressure? According to Mayo Clinic, blood pressure is "the amount of blood your heart pumps and the amount of resistance to blood flow in your arteries" (Mayo Clinic, 2021). When measuring one's blood pressure, two figures (systolic and diastolic) are observed. "The higher number (systolic) represents the pressure while the heart is beating. The lower number (diastolic) represents the pressure when the heart is resting between beats" (Mayo Clinic, 2021). The systolic pressure is always stated first, and the diastolic pressure second (Mayo Clinic, 2021). A normal reading is between 120/80 to 140/90 anything above 140/90 is considered high. However, as of 2017, the American College of Cardiology and the American Heart Association have updated the blood pressure guidelines and a normal reading is now less than 120/80, elevated is between 120-129/80, and stages of hypertension starts at 130/80 (New ACC, 2017).

Having high blood pressure is seen as no big deal, as so many people around the world have it. In fact, in the United States, an estimated 103 million or half of the adult population have high blood pressure (AHA, 2018). The numbers are just as high in the Caribbean and in Jamaica as well. Hypertension affects 21 percent of adults in Barbados and Trinidad and Tobago, between 35 to 38 percent of adults in St. Kitts, British Virgin Islands and Grenada, and 25 percent of adults in Jamaica (Figueroa, 2017). High blood pressure is a risk factor for heart attacks, stroke, and kidney disease and a primary cause of death. In the United States, over 360,000 deaths are a result of high blood pressure (CDC, 2020). While in the Caribbean, it is the cause of 51 percent of deaths from a stroke and 45 percent of deaths from heart disease (Figueroa, 2017).

There are a number of risk factors, such as age, race, family history, being overweight or obese, and health behaviors such as physical inactivity, smoking, and diet that can lead to hypertension. Unfortunately, persons of Black Afro-Caribbean decent are at a greater risk of developing hypertension and especially early in life when compared to other races. Why? Researchers have been unable to determine the exact reason; however, some theories suggest that this is due to higher rates of obesity and diabetes and a gene that was found which makes Blacks more salt-sensitive (AHA, 2016). Additional studies further explained that racial differences exist because Blacks or African Americans, compared to other races, are less likely to engage in physical activity and are disproportionately affected by chronic stressors such as low social economic status, discrimination and relationship stress, and even medication adherence (Munter, 2017).

Based on this information, it seems as if it is not a matter of if someone of the Black race will get hypertension, but when. According to my family's health history, diabetes and glaucoma are prevalent; the only person with high blood pressure that I am aware of is my father. Growing up, I was aware of it but did not know what that even meant. Physically, he looked fine, and I never heard him complain or have physical complications which is probably why it is called the "silent killer." On the other hand, my maternal grandmother had diabetes, and I watched for years as she injected herself with insulin a couple of times a day. She would religiously check her blood sugar and even go into diabetic shock. Year after year, she complained as her health failed. She slowly went blind and eventually had a stroke and died. I saw how she suffered, and every time I would come home from college to visit, she reminded me it would be the last time I would see her. It was difficult for her, and it was difficult for me to see. Naturally, I became concerned about my own risk of developing diabetes but never thought twice about hypertension as I never knew what the typical symptoms or effects "looked" like.

The American Heart Association states that there are no symptoms of high blood pressure. Symptoms such as headaches or even nosebleeds are not caused by high blood pressure. Persons who experience these symptoms might be in hypertensive crisis (which is having a reading above 180/120) or a result of other health conditions (AHA, 2016).

I was first warned about my blood pressure after a routine health check with my gynecologist. He was concerned about my blood pressure and suggested I follow up with a general practitioner for a more comprehensive checkup. I dismissed his recommendation as I had bigger concerns on my plate at the time. I was about to move to Japan. I was young; therefore, I did not need to worry about blood pressure.

Chapter 5 Quotes:

- ❖ "The secret of health for both mind and body is not to mourn for the past, worry about the future, or anticipate troubles but to live in the present." —Buddha
- ❖ "Big journeys begin with the small steps." —Anonymous
- ❖ "Your genetics load the gun. Your lifestyle pulls the trigger." —Mehmet Oz

Chapter 6

Time in the Valley

I saw a sermon online titled, "The Valley is a Temporary Place." The speaker pointed out that we all go through trials and tribulations, crossroads or valley experiences in our lives that we must deal with. There are some experiences that leave us wondering how God could allow this, and some experiences causing uncertainty of how we can even survive. My valley experience happened between the years 2007 to 2011. At the age of twenty-five, I got married, and within less than two months of being married, I found out that my husband was not the person he said he was. I was devastated because this was someone I trusted with my whole heart, and the level of betrayal I received was more than I or anyone who knew about the situation could comprehend. As my friends would say, it was an experience taken straight out of a *Lifetime* movie.

I was so brokenhearted; I did not leave my house for a month; I did not want to answer the phone, and I could not talk to anyone out of fear and humiliation. I was depressed, but I pretended I was fine. I simply accepted it as a typical heartbreak situation and tried to move on. I did not want to deal with the pressure of deciding to divorce or answer any questions about the relationship. I just wanted to run away as far as possible. As a means of escape, I decided to move to Japan. My decision to move to Japan of all places was a light bulb moment. I remembered a conversation I had with a professor my senior year at Ithaca College and her telling me that I should teach English in Japan as an option after graduation. At the time, her suggestion was ridiculous. However, three years later, it felt right. Fortuitously, a few weeks after making the decision to go to Japan I found an ad looking for teachers to come there. I instantly applied and was hired within months.

In the summer of 2008, I packed up my bags and happily moved halfway around the world. My new home was now in Takehara, a small city within the Hiroshima Prefecture. It was the best decision as I loved to travel. I was excited for the change. Before we could start working, we were required to do a health checkup to ensure we were physically capable of handling the job. I was a little apprehensive as I hated going to the doctor. It was a group of us, and I quickly did a scan of everyone and noticed I was the only overweight person in the group. I braced myself to hear that I needed to lose weight. This would be my first experience being called fat in another language. Instead of hearing it verbally, they handed me a piece of paper written in Japanese about my results. I got it translated, and my assumption was correct; my BMI indicated I was morbidly obese; therefore, I was instructed to lose weight along with a few suggestions on how to do so. I was shocked at my weight; I was at my heaviest at this point: 260 pounds. How did I get this big?

I did not focus on addressing my diagnosis; instead, I immersed myself in the culture and everything that Japan had to offer. I was the Assistant Language Teacher (ALT) for four junior high schools; I rotated each of the schools weekly. On weekends, I was free to explore and travel the city. Japan was not a place where you can ever get bored. There were so many museums, festivals and restaurants to visit. I also did not have a car, so public transportation and walking were my main means of getting around. The food was also different; therefore, I started to lose weight within two months of being there.

Japan is a beautiful place, rich in history and tradition, but as a foreigner, I felt lonely. I remember I always wished to be alone, to escape from my family; God heard me and gave me exactly what I asked for, but I sure as hell regretted it. I lived in a studio apartment, and I was the only foreigner and Jamaican in the city. My students were fascinated with me; they were curious about what I ate, the way I looked, and even what I perceived to be normal English language. I was a superstar. Finally, I was getting the attention I always wanted. The Japanese encouraged me to try the local cuisine as much as possible. Though I opened myself up to some of the Japanese cuisine, I gravitated towards what seemed familiar. During my time, it was fun to explore Japan; unfortunately, my previous health diagnosis was starting to catch up with me. I noticed by late 2009 that I started getting frequent headaches; awful, pounding headaches.

One night I was up late and could not sleep. I had cooked dinner and overate and was restless the entire night. While trying to force myself to sleep, I suddenly became aware of my heartbeat, something that does not usually happen unless I am exercising. As I became aware of my heart beating, I recalled once hearing that right before a heart attack, you would have this impending feeling of doom, and I figured, this must be it. I panicked and called 911 immediately. That was not an easy phone call to make. Imagine being afraid and trying to speak a combination of English and Japanese at the same time. I am sure the emergency operators thought I was crazy. Luckily, within a few minutes the ambulance came and transported me to the nearest hospital. They did their tests, and I was fine; it was a panic attack. Over the next year, I had several reoccurrences of the same incident. I was slowly losing my mind because I could not figure out why I was having these panic attacks. Each time was different and slowly got worse; one episode was so bad that my eyesight changed. The doctors ran so many tests, and all indicated that there was nothing physically wrong with me. I wore a 48-hour holster monitor to measure my heart rate, I did a stress test, an echo cardiogram, MRIs, endoscopies, blood tests, and they were all normal.

The doctors tried to explain to me that nothing was wrong. They went through all the tests and said I was physically healthy but diagnosed me as depressed especially based on my frequent visits to the emergency room and 2-night hospital stay. They started me on anti-depressants, which made me feel like I was having an out-of-body experience. I knew I was not clinically depressed but instead felt my concerns were unheard and belittled. Within two weeks, I stopped taking the medication, but the panic attacks continued. The doctor eventually gave me a different kind of medication to take only went I felt anxious. The panic attacks only occurred when I was alone. Therefore, I was so terrified of being alone in my home that I had to ask friends to stay with me or I would visit them every chance I got. I cried when I was alone and barely slept because I feared getting another panic attack.

During this time, I was still in touch with my ex-husband who helped me through the ordeal. He visited me a couple of times in Japan and on those occasions, I never had a panic attack. Unfortunately, the issues between my husband and me that I ignored and tried to escape began to take a toll. He and I started arguing more, and I realized when I began to argue with him, my panic attacks started occurring. This was a totally new development, and I knew I had to sever ties and resolve my health issues to avoid further deterioration.

At this point, I recognized that I needed counseling. I found an English-speaking counselor and had weekly sessions with her. She helped me for a while and she officially diagnosed me with having an anxiety disorder. I knew it was real because when I looked at the list of symptoms, I started having a panic attack; it was that bad. During the weeks that I met with her, I slowly began to open up about my marriage. She was the first person with whom I could openly share exactly how I was feeling without being judged. As a young woman, I believed in marriage and swore that I would never get a divorce and wanted to do all I could to try and save it; but it was becoming too difficult, and I was mentally, emotionally, and physically exhausted.

During this time, I was concerned about my blood pressure as the doctors had informed me that I would probably need to start taking medication, but I needed to start tracking my numbers on my own. I purchased an at-home blood pressure cuff, which was not a good decision for someone with an anxiety disorder. I was anxious while checking my pressure, worried that it would be too high, and instantly visualized the worst. As I saw the readings, I became even more anxious, so I had to stop. After being away from home for almost two years, I came back to Jamaica and spent the summer. This trip took a total of two days, and I was jet-lagged. The day after I got home, I felt so sick; I could not explain the symptoms, but I knew something was wrong. I immediately went to a family doctor, and he checked my blood pressure. He said it was abnormally high, and I needed to be medicated immediately.

The medication worked, so within a few days I started to feel better. After a couple of days of being on the medication it brought my pressure down too low. How did I know? I was at my hair salon, and while getting a manicure I started to see stars; you know when you watch cartoons and you see the character get hit in the head and they see those floating stars? Yes, I started to see those and almost passed out. My mom rushed me to the nearest doctor's office, and my pressure was normal (120/80) by that time. The doctor stopped the medication and determined I was fine to be off medication. I decided to seek a second opinion out of precaution, and I started seeing another doctor who gave me a thorough medical examination and decided that I needed to stay on blood pressure medication for the rest of my life. He determined that I probably had it for a while and did not even know.

While I was home, I slept so much, it was almost as if I had not been sleeping in years. For the first two months I was home, I relaxed and enjoyed my time with family and friends as much as I could. When it was time to go back to Japan, I was so scared; I was terrified of getting sick and having panic attacks again. I eventually got back and still had the panic attacks, but I was able to control them better. The counselor taught me breathing techniques to help cope. Eventually, I made the decision to move back home because I recognized I needed more emotional support that I could not get being so far away. Additionally, I needed to make a decision about my marriage and what I wanted to do long-term. I was back in Jamaica by December 2010.

I made the decision to end my marriage when I moved back to Jamaica. It was not easy, but for my sanity I had to do it. My husband did not take the decision well and had put me through more emotional and mental stress so that I would not leave him. I eventually told him he could only communicate with me through my lawyer because I could not handle it anymore. Over the next year, I filed and waited as the process took its course. During this time, I recognized that I was still suffering from my panic attacks though not as severely. Doing simple tasks like standing in a line at the bank would trigger an attack. Also, I was fearful that my ex-husband would find me. It was ridiculous as he was thousands of miles away in another country, but I knew he would do anything to see me. I was so paranoid of him showing up at my house at any minute that I was even having recurring dreams of tidal waves and tsunamis. In each dream, I would be in a building or somewhere surrounded by water, and eventually, the water would rise and engulf my surroundings, but I would somehow escape. I even dreamt about my husband. In every dream I had of my husband, he would be chasing me or I would be trying to escape from him.

I decided I needed to resume counseling. Over several months, I saw two counselors and they helped me process what was happening. One counselor told me that I was suffering from Post-Traumatic Stress Disorder (PTSD). Usually when we think of PTSD, we associate that with persons who have been in wars or life-endangering situations. She said I should have sought counseling from the very beginning but that was not something I was ready to deal with. She was right; the signs were all there. I did not want to deal with it, and I never knew how to. Eventually, as I discussed my feelings and worked through my emotions, the panic attacks stopped, and I was slowly becoming the newer and improved version of myself.

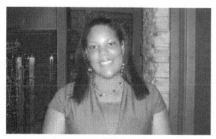
2009
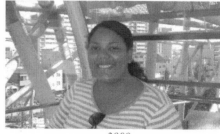
2009

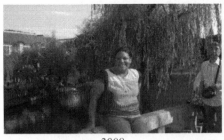
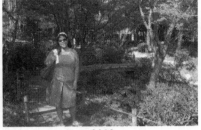

2009   *2009*

Chapter 6 Quotes:

❖ "Be strong now because things will get better. It might be stormy now, but it can't rain forever." —Anonymous

❖ "Sometimes you have to go through the hard times to realize how strong you are." —Anonymous

❖ "Even the darkest night will end, and the sun will rise." — Anonymous

❖ "Keep your head up. God gives his hardest battles to his strongest soldiers." —Anonymous

❖ "Our ability to handle life's challenges is a measure of our strength of character." —Les Brown

Turning Pain into Purpose

While dealing with my emotional and mental well-being, I also had to cope with my new health diagnosis and make significant behavioral changes. Even though I was officially diagnosed with hypertension, I was still eating heavily processed and nutritionally unbalanced meals, but in smaller portions. After making the decision to finally move back to Jamaica in the remaining three months in Japan, I made a conscious effort to change my habits. What I came to appreciate about Japan that aided in my weight loss was the vast differences in the quality and quantity of foods in Japan from western society. For example, in Japan, a loaf of bread only has 6 -10 slices of bread. Similarly, a small-sized drink in western culture equates to a large size drink in Japan. Even the sugar and fat content in foods are significantly less in sweet treats such as ice cream and cakes. In addition, while dining out in restaurants in Japan, the complimentary starter is not a warm basket of bread or salty crispy chips or something battered up and fried, but simply vegetables. In fact, all meals in Japan always had some form of fruit or vegetables. These slight differences aided in my weight loss. Between September 2008 to August 2010, I went from 260 pounds to 200 pounds. After my diagnosis, I had to do an overdue assessment of my eating habits.

My diagnosis of being hypertensive was not easy as I came to the realization that my health was now dependent on pills. I hate taking pills. I only took pills when it was necessary, and on those occasions, I always asked for the liquid alternative. If I had no choice but to take tablets, I would crush it or take the ingredients out of the capsule. I viewed pills as a temporary fix; now I was sentenced to taking medications for the rest of my life.

At first, I was prescribed one pill daily. It took some adjustment to remember to take it. Some days I forgot and threw the pills away by accident. Eventually, I got the hang of it. It also took some time to find the right dosage and brand that worked with my body. I dealt with a number of unpleasant side effects. One brand caused an allergic reaction as I broke out in hives. With other brands I felt nauseated, had heart palpitations, and experienced fatigue and worst of all, my blood pressure was not well regulated. Eventually, my doctor placed me on three different medications at high doses. I was not happy, but that also showed the severity of my condition.

Being labeled as hypertensive and having to share my new health status and medical history was just frustrating. Doctors were shocked and dumbfounded that someone so young was suffering from this diagnosis. I was overwhelmed by the numerous doctor visits and tests; I just wanted everything to be normal again. From this point, I did not care about how I looked anymore but rather about becoming healthy and what I had to do to reverse this disease. I was on a mission. I began searching on the internet for natural remedies to lower blood pressure. I educated myself on the effects of sodium in the body and how much sodium our bodies actually need. I found the *Dash Diet,* which is a healthy eating approach to lowering blood pressure. I eliminated salt completely and started cutting out processed foods one by one and replacing them with wholesome alternatives. For example, for breakfast I usually ate cereals, pancakes or omelets filled with cheese and toasted bread with butter. I switched to granola with milk and then to flavored prepackaged instant oatmeal. As I became more educated about foods and reading nutritional labels, I made further adjustments. A key example was moving from processed instant oatmeal with high sugar content to unflavored old fashion oatmeal sweetened with fruits. Making these types of dietary changes did not feel restrictive or difficult but made me feel in control for the first time in a long while. In conjunction, I increased and became more consistent with exercise and started seeing losing the weight effortlessly. I finally had the power to improve my health in a way that felt right.

When I moved back to Jamaica in December of 2010, I was down to 180 pounds. The entire process for me was not about reducing my weight out of vanity or to please someone else; this was about changing my life completely and making healthier decisions that would be sustainable. By the time I settled in at home and began a routine, I was militant about everything I placed in my body. I was open to new and healthy recipes, eating more salads, and even eating vegan options. When I would dine in at restaurants, I requested all meals to be sodium-free and started drinking freshly made vegetable juices. In the past the thought of a vegetable as a drink was repulsive; it was "lawn in a bowl." Now eating this way has become a regular part of my daily life.

By the end of 2011, I lost a little over 100 pounds in total. In January 2012, I decided to be brave and share my story with the *All Woman* column in the Jamaica Observer newspaper. At the time, the column was looking for persons who had lost a significant amount of weight to share their stories. I did it because it took me years to get to this point, and unfortunately, I was one of those persons who became afflicted with a lifestyle disease in order to take my health seriously. At the time I was featured in the article, I was 155 pounds, but my goal was 147 pounds and to be a size eight. By the summer of 2012, I successfully accomplished my goal. I was now the same size as my mother; I was shocked.

I was getting compliments constantly from those who knew me; some people could not recognize me because I did not look the same. Persons even exclaimed that I was getting too skinny and that I should "stop losing weight now; you're wasting away." Comments like those made me realize you can never please people. When you are fat, there is a problem, and when you lose the weight, that's another problem. At this point, I did not care what anyone said. I cared about how I felt, and I felt amazing. Physically, yes, I finally felt comfortable in my skin.

Having lost all the weight, I was happy to go shopping again. I could now go into any "normal" store, like Express or H&M, and feel confident that something would finally fit me. I did not cringe when I looked in the mirror and saw the person staring back at me. I was shocked at who I was now. It took me a while to accept the new me. My friends could tell I struggled with becoming the new version of Stacy and voiced that I still carried myself as a fat person; the inside needed to match the outside. Apparently, the damage from the years of negativity and self-hate needed some more time to catch up to the new me.

A number of persons say that when they lose weight, certain physical ailments disappear, like sleep apnea, skin issues, or breathing problems. Thankfully, even when I was heavier I did not have any physical complications. Obvious changes could be seen in my face; the shape of my head went from round to a more elongated shape, and my nose was less pudgy. My eyes, in particular, changed as when I used to smile, the fat around my face would squeeze my eyes shut because I was so big. I have loose skin on my arms, stomach, breasts, and legs. It is not nearly as bad having lost over 100 pounds, but it is there. My feet have also shrunken. I went from a size 10 down to 8 or 8.5 in shoes. Most importantly, my blood pressure was under control. I still had to deal with various side effects, which I complained to my doctor every chance I got, but I was learning to deal with them. The side effects made me more vigilant in wanting to get off medication as quickly as possible. My doctor reminded me that I needed to take time with this process, and I should not be too quick to get off the medication. As of 2012, I was on three medications. I begged my doctor to reduce me to two just to see how I would do, and it worked. I was officially down to two medications.

Now that I had reached my targeted size and weight, I needed to maintain the weight loss to ensure and avoid going back to who I was before. I became so afraid of going back to the old me because I did not want to undo everything I had achieved; I did not want to become sick again.

My newfound passion in health education inspired me to pursue my master's degree in public health and therefore migrated to the United States in 2013. I was excited, yet afraid especially because of the types of food, change in environment, and the change in routine and how it would undo everything I worked so hard for. Life as a student posed its challenges: hectic schedule and limited resources. In my first year, I did wonderfully. I ensured I made healthy choices. Every meal had some form of vegetable or protein. If I had to eat foods from restaurants or catered foods, I chose the healthiest option. As a student, the fitness center was always at my disposal, so I made sure to include exercise in my schedule. I did not allow time, assignments, or the cold bitter winters to stop me from exercise; I went no matter what. As a result, I lost even more weight. I had gotten down to a size 6, and as a bonus, the doctor who was managing my health in the US lowered one of my medications by one full dosage.

Did I ever slip back into old eating habits of eating processed and junk foods? Yes. Did I regain some weight? Of course. In 2015, the final year in the masters program, I was consumed with finishing my courses, studying for my certification exam, completing my internship, and working. The days and nights were long, and I was less focused on my eating habits. However, I never got too out of control; I still exercised and ate balanced meals, but I was not as concerned. I think I allowed myself to be more carefree because I felt more in control and started feeling I should even regain some weight (What was I thinking?) By the time I graduated in August 2015 to February 2016, I gained ten pounds. After working for one year, I moved back to Jamaica in October 2016 and weighed one hundred and sixty-nine pounds.

How did I manage to regain so much weight in a short span of time? Honestly, there were many factors, but if I think about it, I was living again and reached a point where I had other things going for me. I was healthy, my blood pressure was still consistently under control, and I stopped thinking about it. I stopped focusing on my life-long goal of being off medication completely. I was more concerned with my career and job placement. By the time I moved back to Jamaica, it was then I realized how much weight I had regained. Now twenty-two pounds in the grand scheme of things is not a big deal, per say. My doctors were not concerned; my blood pressure was still under control, blood tests showed everything was still normal, but I felt like I had let myself down. I still received compliments about how I looked. My family said I looked "healthier" again, but I felt uncomfortable. I was not sad or depressed; I did not allow myself to eat my way back into a size 18; I simply felt uncomfortable. So, I did something about it.

One thing I have come to realize is that life is ever evolving; what worked before will not necessarily work again. I am older now, and my metabolism may not necessarily be the same. As women, we have so many hormones that can affect our bodies, even foods that we could eat when we were younger, we can no longer tolerate when we reach a certain age group. Now for me, I did not have any hormonal imbalances going on; I still needed to educate myself more and figure out what was working and what was not. I am by no means an expert on all things regarding health. Up to this point, I educated myself on the importance of eating whole foods and less processed foods and the nutrients needed to maintain a healthy blood pressure.

Thanks to the internet and social media, there is so much information from across the world. I managed to learn from different health coaches and healthy lifestyle advocates on the importance of meal planning and incorporating more healthy foods into my daily life and being aware of emotional eating and things that we do not think about that can impact our health. Within a few months, I lost 12 pounds.

Since 2017, I have been maintaining a weight of 155. In 2013, my doctor overseas reduced my medication, and since then, it has been reduced to about another full dosage here in Jamaica. As of 2018, my current doctor is working with me to lower it even more and eventually get me off medication completely. She reminds me that as I get older, I may have to go back on it, but I am happy about my progress. Having reached my goal, I have other goals in mind, as there is still work that needs to be done. My new goal is not focused per say on losing weight but more on adding tone and definition to my body. In order to lose weight, I was not focused on strength training but on cardio. Not incorporating strength training could be the result of my loose skin or could be a result of how much my skin has stretched. Either way, I am now learning to do more strength training and thinking about doing exercises that result in more muscles. I will be the first one to tell you I dislike strength training; I find it monotonous, but it is what I need to do in order to achieve my next goal.

My quest for health has definitely taken longer than I thought, but it has taught me the importance of resilience and persistence, knowing your body, and fighting for yourself. It is never too late, and it is about finding out what works for you.

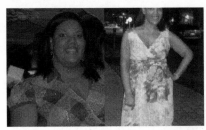

2008 vs. 2015

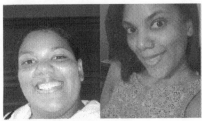

2008 vs. 2021

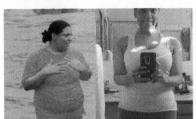

2004 vs. 2020

Chapter 7 Quotes:

* ❖ "Dreams come true if you survive the hard times." — Anonymous
* ❖ "Sometimes the bad things that happen in our lives put us directly on the path to the best things that will ever happen to us." —Nicole Reed

❖ "Until you're broken, you don't know what you're made of. It gives you the ability to build yourself again, but stronger than ever." —Anonymous

❖ "For God hath not given us the spirit of fear; but of power, and of love, and of a sound mind." —2 Timothy 1:7 (KJV)

Chapter 8

Practical Strategies about Eating Right

Many of you may have realized that this is not a diet or how to lose weight fast type of book. My focus from this point onwards will be additional strategies that worked for me and how you can utilize them. Before starting any diet or exercise routine, always consult a medical professional like your doctor, nurse, or nutritionist.

Have you ever noticed when you start a diet, how restricted and hungry you feel, and find yourself counting down the days, minutes, and seconds to when you can have that piece of bread or even eat a piece of fruit? This way of eating is not sustainable long term unless your goal is to lose a few pounds due to a "snack accident" or vacation overindulgence; then, do what is best for you. The following suggestions may not be for you. The following strategies are for persons who need and want to make life-long changes.

1. ***Keep a diary or food journal of what you eat.*** Try this for just one week so you can have an idea of the types of foods (even counting those foods you are just sampling count too) you are putting in your body and the number of calories you are consuming daily. By doing this, you have a visual representation of what's causing you to gain weight. You will also be able to identify the foods you are allergic to and

those that are making you sick. The point of this activity is to not make you feel guilty but to empower you to take control of your eating habits.

2. ***Alternate/swap unhealthy foods for healthier foods.*** Living a healthy lifestyle should not be difficult, dieting is. Dieting is almost like self-punishment and reinforces the notion that foods are bad. Instead, we should be able to enjoy those foods we love in moderation but also have healthier alternatives. Have you ever heard of the concept called "*Eat This, Not That*"? Do just that, pick the healthier option. For example, I love eating pasta, but instead of eating the regular white pasta, I eat whole wheat instead. It has more fiber, less carbohydrates, and more vitamins and minerals. Nowadays, there are so many kinds of pastas that could suit your health needs. Do you love rice? Try brown rice or quinoa; you can even mix them. You can even try cauliflower rice; it is actually pretty good. With regard to sodas and juices, find ones with reduced sugar, or juices that are natural as much as possible; the less added sugar the better.

Try making healthy swaps with your condiments as well. For example, instead of mayonnaise, use Greek yogurt; they even have vegan mayonnaise or vegan yogurts as well. I love making mashed potatoes sometimes, so instead of using milk or butter, I may add Greek yogurt, and it is super creamy and delicious. Avocado is another great substitute for butter. An avocado contains "good" fat that is high in potassium and other vitamins and minerals. There are also a number of snack options that can be healthy and satisfy those cravings we all get. Instead of chips, try nuts (almonds, pumpkin seeds). I love nuts: almonds, cashews, peanuts, I love them all. I buy them raw and unsalted; that way I can roast them myself. If I get the salted kind, I wash the salt off (Really!) Allergic to nuts but still want chips, make your own.

By making these switches, you are reducing your intake of overly processed high saturated fats, excess sugar, and empty calories for foods that have the necessary vitamins and minerals that our bodies need. You should feel better and ultimately lose weight. However, as a warning, do not overindulge. Some of these healthy options are high in calories and fat so remember moderation and portion control are important too.

3. *Read food labels.* A lot of people do not take the time to read labels because it is time consuming and difficult, but it is not. If you find it a waste of time, then I implore you to shop for foods that do not come with a label. Honestly, in the past, I could not tell you the kind of information that is found on a food label except for the ingredients. In fact, I did not care at all. After being diagnosed with hypertension, I actually saw how much salt, sugars, fats, and calories I was consuming thoughtlessly. This was an eye-opener. The images below are illustrations of a food label. You will notice two labels, the *original label* and the *new label*. Both labels provide the same nutritional information; however, the *new label* has been updated with an easy-to-read design to help consumers make informed food choices. Why the change? According to the Food and Drug Administration (FDA), the new label is "consistent with current data on the associations between nutrients and chronic diseases, health-related conditions…as well as consumer understanding and consumption patterns" (FDA, 2016). As you will notice, there are updates to the font size and display of the

information. However, the biggest amendment has been the added sugars. The original label listed the total sugars, while the new label shows the natural sugar and how much sugar has been added during the processing of the food.

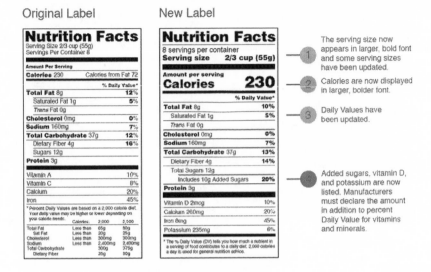

Source: Overlake Medical Center & Clinics. (June 2, 2020). How to Read the 2020 Nutrition Labels. Retrieved from https://www.overlakehospital.org/blog/how-read-2020-nutrition-labels

Reading food labels helps us see the serving size and caloric intake to make more informed decisions as well as awareness around certain nutritional factors such as sugars, saturated fat, and sodium. When looking at a label for the first time, do not become overwhelmed; try looking at it categorically. Which means, what nutrients do you need more of, and what things should you avoid or limit? Therefore, if you are hypertensive, you need to limit your sodium or salt intake while consuming more potassium. Reading food labels takes practice, be patient. If you are in a rush and do not have time to read while shopping, do your research before leaving home. This will reduce the amount of time you spend in the supermarket or grocery store.

4. **_Drink more water._** We have all heard before that we need to drink more water, and you will hear it again here too. Drinking water is important for your body as it keeps your body temperature normal, helps to lubricate and cushion your joints, and gets rid of bodily wastes through urination, perspiration, and bowel movements (CDC, 2021). How much water do you need in a day? Typically, we have all heard eight glasses of water daily; however, the actual amount varies based on a number of factors. For example, if you live in warmer countries like Jamaica, you will need more. If you are physically active, work or playing outdoors, you will need to drink more as well. Even having certain health conditions, as well as being pregnant and-or breastfeeding makes it important to drink lots of water.

Do not wait until you are thirsty to actually drink water; if you do, that means your body is already dehydrated. You know how hydrated you are based on the color of your urine. If it is colorless to light yellow, you are properly hydrated. If it is difficult to drink lots of water because you either do not like it or based on your environment, then try to get water when having your meals or when taking a break. Bring a water bottle with you, which is a great reminder to drink water. If you must buy water, avoid those with added flavors. The nutritional labels will show that some have added sugars. If you need to drink your water with something to take away the bland and boring taste, add your own flavors from fruits like lime or lemon, strawberries, orange slices, and even cucumbers. You can also increase your water intake by "eating." There are lots of fruits and vegetables that have a high water content like cucumbers, iceberg lettuce, melons, celery, oranges, tomatoes, grapefruit, and coconuts.

5. ***Reduce sodium intake/eliminate added salt.*** We often hear salt and sodium being used interchangeably; they are different. Sodium is an important mineral that occurs naturally in foods, while salt or table salt is a combination of sodium and chloride. Sodium is essential for our bodies. It is controlled by our kidneys, and it helps to control the body's fluid balance. Sodium also aids in sending nerve impulses and affects muscle function. It can be found in canned or prepared foods like processed meats and frozen dinners. The American Heart Association says that over 70 percent of the sodium we eat comes from processed, pre-packaged and restaurants foods, while the remaining comes from naturally occurring foods and what is added when cooking and eating (AHA, 2018). Based on this, we are eating way more salt than is recommended. In fact, most people consume about 3,400 milligrams in a day (Nutrition, 2021). It is recommended by the American Heart Association that we eat no more than 2,399 milligrams (1 teaspoon) of sodium in a day or ideally no more than 1,500 milligrams (½ teaspoon) (AHA, 2018). How can we do that? Read your food labels (See no. 3). Look at the amount of sodium content when buying packaged, frozen, and canned foods. If you choose these items, go for the ones that have reduced sodium, less sodium, or no added salt.

Cook without salt; I know that is really difficult but try adding herbs, seasonings and spices for flavoring instead. When dining out, tell restaurants not to add salt if possible or choose items low in sodium. What has worked for me is, if I know I am going to a restaurant and I may want to splurge and have a good time, I ensure that the sodium in the other two meals for the day was very limited. Even with that in mind, I do not go overboard at restaurants. The American Heart Association's website, www.heart.org, has additional tips on how to reduce sodium intake.

6. *Eat/drink less sugar.* In the same way that sodium naturally occurs in foods, so does sugar in foods like fruit and milk. Processed sugars like corn syrup, other syrups and white and brown sugar are the ones that we need to reduce and eliminate from our diet. These are unnecessary calories that will start a chain reaction to a bunch of things we do not want, such as weight gain and various diseases. The maximum amount of added sugar that should be consumed in a day is 25 grams or 6 teaspoons for women, and 37.5 grams or 9 teaspoons for men (Gunnars, 2021). When I first heard that, I thought it actually sounds like a lot, but it is not. I love chocolate milk (do not judge me), particularly the 14oz Nesquik low-fat double chocolate milk drink. The amount of sugar is 38 grams per serving. That one drink contains my entire day's serving of sugar and more. Sodas and fruit juices are all the same, which is why it is important to read the labels and reduce the amount we consume. How? By trying to avoid these drinks like the plague. If you have been drinking a lot of soda and juices for a while, it may be difficult to just cut them out completely. Slowly start to wean yourself off. For example, if you know you drink two bottles of soda a day, try and cut it down to once per day. Then, the following week, drink a diet soda and eventually start replacing soda with water. If you are not a soda drinker but love juice (like myself), substitute it with water or eat the whole fruit instead of juice. The whole fruit has fiber

which makes you feel fuller. Try as best as possible to cut out baked goods, cookies, cakes, and sweets. What works for me is not having the item that causes me temptation in my house at all. I know what my weaknesses are, so if I can help it, I do not bring them home. If the craving hits me, I try to satisfy it with a better option. Or, I give into the craving and enjoy the baked good occasionally. Right now, it is Easter, and in Jamaica, it is the season for bun and cheese. For those of you who do not know, bun is a highly spiced bread with lots of fruits, raisins, and a truckload of sugar. It is found all year round, but the demand is higher around this time of year. For something like this, it is good to consume as little as possible, especially if you eat it regularly. Again, read the food labels and observe the sugar content. Just because it says reduced or less calories does not mean it is not high in sugar. Let us be real as well, we all have cravings for these "bad" foods. If you can completely avoid these sweet items, more power to you, do just that. If you love it, enjoy it in moderation.

7. *Eat more fruits and vegetables*. One thing that has helped me tremendously is instead of worrying about what not to eat or what to avoid, I try to think about what I should eat more of. We should be consuming four and five servings of fruits and vegetables respectively (US Department of Health and Human Services, n.d.). The easiest way to do that is to ensure that every meal has a serving of each. To ensure that we get enough of each should not be complicated. The following illustration is a great way to remind us, instead of having to actually measure every single item.

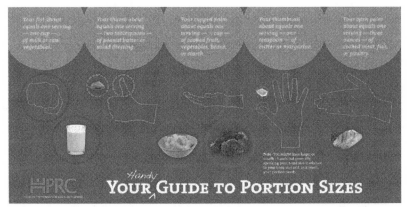

YOUR GUIDE TO PORTION SIZES

Source: Human Performance Resources (n.d.). How to gauge food portion sizes. Retrieved from: https://www.hprc-online.org/articles/how-to-gauge-food-portion-sizes

I have developed a love for drinking fresh vegetable juices and smoothies and eating vegetarian or vegan meals, which aids in getting the recommended servings I need daily. There are so many movements encouraging, motivating, and helping us to eat properly, for example, "Vegan" or "Meatless" Mondays, where you dedicate that one day to eating only fruits and vegetables. It is great to try these things out; they can be fun and open your palette to healthy eating that does not have to be boring. In Jamaica, there are tons of restaurants that are vegan, that have transformed fruits and vegetables into tasteful dishes. Some restaurants in Jamaica that I love are New Leaf Restaurant and Tehuti Café. I also follow a number of persons on social media who give me ideas on recipes to try.

8. ***Physical Activity.*** In the next chapter, I will provide more details about this. Part of a healthy lifestyle is getting exercise or being physically active (I will use these words interchangeably). Physical activity works in tandem with your eating habits.

9. ***Be careful when dining out.*** Most restaurants (in the United States) show the caloric amount and or the ingredients in the foods they serve, which makes it easier to choose the healthier option. In some cases, the healthy option does not always mean it is actually healthy. For example, a salad smothered in dressing with tons of cheese and toppings coated in sugar and fats is just as bad as a cheeseburger. When dining out, most restaurants can and will cater to your needs; it is just a matter of asking. For example, you can ask for your food to not have added salt. I have been to a variety of restaurants that happily accommodate my request. They will explain if the item is pre-prepared with certain seasonings, so they either do not add additional salt or leave the specific seasoning with salt completely off. If salt cannot be removed from the requested item, they may suggest another option. If I really want my chosen item, I ensure the side items, like the cooked vegetables, are salt-free.

    I love drinking protein shakes and smoothies as well; some places may add sweeteners like honey or cane juice for additional sweetness. Unfortunately, some neglect to list these add-ons on their menu; it is only while observing them that you may find out. Therefore, ensure you ask and ask for it to be taken out. I do that because I have grown accustomed to eating so many things without sugar that I do not need it; you may be surprised to see it is already sweet without it.

10. ***Change your environment.*** Want to live a long healthy life? Change your environment. To assist with the changes in your lifestyle, your environment must reflect that as well (Nania, 2017). For example, if your goal is to drink more water, buy a reusable water bottle that you can carry with you when you are on the go. Place the water bottle in eye

view or have it close by as a reminder. If your goal is to eat more fruits, you should place them somewhere within your home (kitchen) that you can see them. According to one research study out of Cornell University, keeping unhealthy foods out of sight and having healthy foods easily visible had a big impact on the test subjects' weight (Ahn 2014). The overall point is to ensure that you make adjustments where possible to your environment so that it is easier to adopt healthier choices.

11. **Meal prep.** Meal prepping is a huge lifesaver. When I have prepared for the week, I do not have to worry about what to eat, and I am less likely to eat carelessly. It is best to try and find one day out of the week where you can cook everything in that day to store and refrigerate for the next few days or week. For me, I cook on Sundays and pack into containers the meals for lunch, so I simply reheat at lunchtime. I will also cook a big pot of soup and have that at dinnertime. If I made too much, I freeze and defrost it whenever I feel for it again. Some foods you may want fresh, so for smoothies and juices, you can cut up the items and store them in individual serving sizes. When you are ready, just take it out and blend. Just doing those simple preparations ahead of time helps to cut down on time in some way. For my vegetables, I try to juice them for days in advance and store them in air-tight containers. This helps preserve the nutrients and cuts down on me cleaning a juicer or blender daily. If you do not want to prepare for an entire week, just do a few days and do what works best for you.

12. **Portion Control:** I spoke about this briefly, but I decided I needed to say it again, especially if you want to lose or maintain weight. It is something you must be aware of when

you are dining at home or out but more so when eating out. If you look at foods today, they are almost double the size of what they used to be a few years ago.

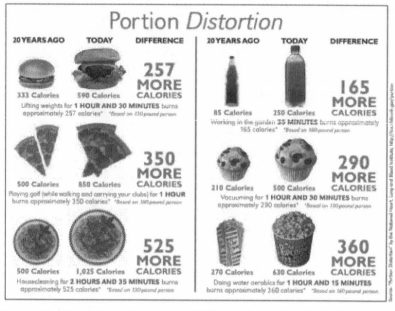

Source: Positive Choice Integrative Wellness Center (Jan 7, 2019). Portion vs. Serving Size. Retrieved from: https://positivechoice.org/portion-vs-serving-size/

The above picture is an example of how the size of the everyday foods we consume has changed over the past twenty years. Obviously, the foods are bigger and contain more calories, which means we are eating more than we should. This is one of the reasons behind weight gain. Now, I will agree you have no control over how much the food industry serves us; however, just because they gave it to you does not mean you need to eat it all in one sitting. Instead of eating the entire muffin, have half and save the other half for the next day. Sometimes you may not have the option of saving things for later. If that is the case, eat less at your next meal. In Jamaica, for example, boxed lunches are very popular; these are hot lunches of rice with some meat (like curry goat and rice, fried chicken with curry gravy and rice, just to name a few). Boxed lunches are filled with what seems like almost a pound of rice with tons of gravy and maybe a couple of pieces of meat. From the looks of one carton, it could be two meals. Some people eat like this daily and cannot understand why they are struggling with their weight. So, if your goal is to lose weight, a good place to start is by trying to reduce your portion sizes. Try to eat half of what you normally get and save the rest for later or the next day's meal (good way to save money too). If you can, ask for less rice and add more vegetables when possible.

13. ***Consult nutritionist/dietitian.*** Above I mentioned a lot of points on reducing your intake of sugar, saturated fats, and sodium, but if you feel you need the help of a professional to better guide you, I definitely recommend that. They have the expertise to guide you on how many calories you need to consume to reach your goals and what food combinations work for you based on your individual needs.

14. ***Be patient and forgive yourself.*** If you forget everything else, I hope you will remember to exercise patience and forgiveness towards yourself. Unlearning, relearning, and retraining your brain is a process that takes time. A lot of the things I have mentioned did not happen overnight, and I am sure I have tons more to learn. I have made mistakes (a lot of them) and have failed to follow my own advice a number of times. I sometimes drank my chocolate milk even though I had juice on the same day; I have forgotten to tell the waiter or waitress to hold the salt; I have had the full-fat dressing with sugar; I have eaten processed foods instead of a healthier alternative because I had a stressful week and was

too exhausted to care, and the list goes on. I feel guilty, of course, but I remind myself that I am human, that life is short, and I can live a little, and there are plenty of other days where I will get it right. Remember, as long as there is life, you have another chance to make better decisions.

Chapter 8 Quotes:

- ❖ "Weight loss doesn't begin on the gym with a dumbbell; it starts in your head with a decision." —Toni Sorenson
- ❖ "Healthy habits are learned in the same way as unhealthy ones—through practice." —Wayne Dyer
- ❖ "Small daily improvements are the key to long-term staggering results." —Anonymous
- ❖ "It's all about creating healthy habits, not restrictions." — Anonymous

Chapter 9

Living Right

E ating right is very important if you want to live a healthy lifestyle or lose weight. However, exercise is another important piece of the puzzle. Many persons do not exercise for a number of reasons, ranging from having physical injuries, a busy schedule, lack of energy, and just hate to exercise. Having an exercise routine does not have to be overly complicated or militant. There are many forms and types of workouts that can be completed, depending on your goals and level of fitness.

Types of Exercise

Aerobic (Cardio) Exercises: This is a continuous activity that works your heart, lungs, and muscles. This type of exercise improves your cardiovascular and endurance levels; it is ideal for weight loss and weight maintenance (Bupa UK, n.d.). Examples of this type of exercise are:

- Walking
- Cycling
- Running/jogging
- Swimming
- Sports (tennis, football, basketball)

- Aerobic machines (treadmills, elliptical, spinning bikes) (Bupa UK, n.d.).

Strength Exercises: This type of exercise focuses on building and/or maintaining the strength of your muscles. It aids in the development of "muscle strength and healthy bones in childhood, and to maintain these as an adult. In later life, strengthening exercises help to delay the natural decline in muscle mass and bone strength." (Bupa UK, n.d.). Examples of this type of exercise are:

- Resistance bands
- Weights
- Resistance machines
- Gardening/shopping (lifting heavy, everyday items or using our own body weight) (Bupa UK, n.d.)

Flexibility Exercises: This type of exercise improves your flexibility and can help keep you mobile and active (Bupa UK, n.d.). It involves stretching your body into various positions. This helps with strength, balance, and relaxation. Examples of this type of exercise are:

- Yoga
- Pilates (Bupa UK, n.d.)

Balancing Exercises: This is a type of exercise that aids in mobility and balance (Bupa UK, n.d.). It helps reduce your risk of falling as you get older. Examples of this type of exercise are:

- Dancing
- Tai chi
- Tennis

- Standing on one leg
- Walking backwards
- Walking on your toes
- Calf raises
- Toe raises (Bupa UK, n.d.)

As you have just read, exercising does not have to be only going to the gym or a physical location and using a treadmill. Exercise is walking, climbing stairs, doing chores, gardening, even walking around in a mall. For example, I went on vacation for two weeks in 2018, and every day I took the subway or went walking the streets of Philadelphia, site seeing, hanging with friends, and shopping; I did not sweat or exert myself in any way. For several hours a day, I just walked, and by the time my vacation was over, I was five pounds lighter. Utilizing your home or work environment can be very beneficial for those with busy schedules and limited time to dedicate 30 to 60 minutes consecutively. You can break up 30 minutes into five or 10-minute intervals in an 8-hour day. For example, take the stairs only while at the office. No stairs on the job, then use whatever you have at your disposal. It can be as simple as occasionally walking to your colleague to speak to them instead of calling or completing stretches right at your desk. Be creative. For those who work from home and/or have children to take care of, you can also use your environment to your advantage. Have errands on the road? When you stop at any location, park your car at a further distance away from the store to get additional daily steps. If the options are between an escalator and the stairs, take the stairs instead. Even the stairs in your home will provide the cardio to get your heart pumping.

My point is, start small, start where you feel comfortable, and start with what you have and can afford. If you have never exercised a day in your life and you are a beginner or you have certain medical conditions or physical limitations, first and foremost, get your doctor's or health provider's approval. Once cleared, start with their recommendation. When I was heavier, I was terrified of going to certain fitness centers because everybody looked physically in shape and I felt intimidated. You want to be in a place that motivates and supports you and does not care about how you look. If you cannot afford to go to the gym because it is just not in the budget, go walking instead. In Jamaica, for example, many walk or cycle around the neighborhoods or in parks. I was unemployed for months, even up to two years, so I could not afford the gym. I did not allow that to stop me from exercising. I walked around my neighborhood. No interest in doing it alone? Grab a friend or a family member. This can be a great time to catch up and burn calories. Do not want to leave the house just yet? There are numerous videos for every fitness level. Remember, something is better than nothing.

No matter what you do, there are many benefits to exercise. Such as:

1. Losing weight
2. Maintaining weight
3. Preventing and managing health conditions and diseases (that is, high blood pressure, type 2 diabetes, bad cholesterol, depression, anxiety, and cancer)
4. Improving your mood
5. Boosting energy
6. Promoting better sleep
7. Improving your sex life (MayoClinc, 2019)

How Much Physical Activity Do we Need?

General health benefits:

The World Health Organization recommends for adults between the ages of 18-64 years old, 150 minutes weekly (30 minutes, 5 times per week) of moderate intense aerobic physical activity plus strength training (WHO, n.d.). Strength training is just as important as a cardio workout. In fact, we should be incorporating it into our physical activity sessions. Why? Well, cardio helps us burn calories, which makes us lose weight according to fitness experts. However, strength training helps us get stronger, leaner, and burns calories longer. The American Heart Association recommends adults do strength training at least twice weekly (AHA, n.d.). The level of intensity, the type and the duration of the exercise are based on your goals.

Prevent Weight Gain and Active Weight Loss:

150-200 (40 minutes, 5 times per week) minutes per week
150-300 (60 minutes, 5 times per week) minutes per week

Prevention of Weight Regain:

200-300 (60 minutes, 5 times per week) minutes per week
300-400 (80 minutes, 5 times per week) minutes per week

Maintain your Weight:

150 (30 minutes, 5 times per week) per week (AHA, n.d.)

I tried to go to the gym 4-6 days weekly; I used the treadmill and attended aerobic classes and did some strength training. Zumba, spinning, and kickboxing were some of my favorite classes. I really worked up a good sweat and rid my body of the fatigue and stress of the day. Strength training is something I have to push myself to do because I find it so monotonous. During my weight loss, I focused solely on cardio exercises, and because of that, I do not have a lot of muscles; I am now trying to focus more on toning and increasing my muscle mass. Health experts recommend that we do strength exercises at least two times weekly (Bupa UK, n.d.).

Getting physical exercise and going to the gym is great, but I do not always feel motivated to go. I have my moments where I make excuses, such as cramps because of my menstruation cycle, I had a rough day at work, the cold, the flu, it's raining, the traffic on the road looks bad or, plain and simple, I just do not want to go. If I have those days, I try not to let more than one day pass too often, but there have been occasions where I skipped the gym for weeks or even months. I felt guilty, but I got over it and went right back at it again. I always remember that euphoric feeling I get every time I have completed a workout, and that helps me to not miss the gym for long periods of time.

Consistency is very important, and we all have moments where we will miss a day or two of getting some form of physical activity, but do not let it become a habit or allow it to get out of control. When I have those moments of laziness, fatigue, I do not allow my thoughts to dwell on how I feel; I push myself and go anyway. Sometimes my energy is so low when I start my aerobics class or when I am on the treadmill, but after a few minutes, I feel invigorated and energized and happy I made the right decision.

What is the reason behind becoming healthy or getting exercise? For me, I focused on my blood pressure more so than my weight. I thought about all that I had been through to get to this very point to help me stay on track. Therefore, I encourage you to use whatever reasons you have to push yourself and help you stay the course. If you do not see the physical progress right away, do not give up. Do not focus solely on the number on the scale but on how you feel and other non-scale achievements like how your clothes fit, your energy, better sleep, improved performance, etc. I promise you, the scale will eventually budge. If it still doesn't move or goes in the wrong direction, throw that sucker away. Progress can be measured in more ways than one; you are more than the number on the scale.

When is the Best Time to Exercise?

When implementing an exercise program into your schedule, you may wonder if there is an ideal time. In fact, there is research on the benefits and challenges or pros and cons with morning and evening workout sessions. Here is a list:

Benefits	
Morning	**Evening**
Increases energy level in the afternoon	Bodily functions at its highest/More energy and more strength for an optimal workout
Helps burn fat more effectively	
	Muscles and joints more flexible/Less strain to exercise and less chance of injuries
Increased metabolism (burns calories throughout the day)	
	More energy/More strength and endurance
Improved sleep at night	Outlet for stress

Less chance of missing a workout (fewer schedule conflicts)	Better for maximal anaerobic leg exercises
Get it done and out the way. You have the rest of day to do other things	More strength
Best time for cardio if you want to lose weight	Burn less fat

Challenges	
Morning	**Evening**
Less time to sleep in late/Less motivated to wake up early	Working out too close to bedtime could make it more difficult to fall asleep.
Less strength	
	More likely to skip exercise after a long workday
Joints and muscles are stiffer at awakening, so you are more prone to injuries	
	More crowds at the gym
Exercising before breakfast increases the risk of burnout and fatigue	
	More chances of work activities occurring

Adapted from AIA at https://www.aia.com.my/en/what-matters/health-wellness/morning-vs-evening-workouts--which-is-better-.html

There are countless studies that have shown the differences in physical performance when exercises are completed in the morning versus the afternoon. I could share them, but honestly, unless you are an athlete in training, it is irrelevant. What I will say is, the best time to work out is based on your schedule. For years, I was a huge advocate for working out in the evenings because I was not a fan of waking up early; at 5 am or even 6 am, it is still so dark out, with a warm comfortable bed that wants me to stay even longer. Even with an alarm, I would hit snooze every five minutes; pissed that every minute felt like seconds, I would eventually turn it off, give in and say, "maybe I'll work out later or tomorrow." Sometimes, later or tomorrow never happened.

As I mentioned earlier, I loved classes like Zumba and spinning. I found that those classes were commonly offered early in the morning. Occasionally, I would force myself to wake up early once per week so I could go to those classes because of how much I enjoyed them. I eventually stopped because I gave into my feelings of not wanting to wake up early. Therefore, I stuck with my evening workouts. Life is always evolving, and we must learn to adapt to those changes especially if our health depends on it.

Change Your Routine According To Schedule

Fast forward to 2021, I have found myself appreciating and loving morning workouts. In 2020, I got a job with the Ministry of Health and Wellness right before the COVID-19 pandemic hit Jamaica. There were a number of days that required long hours, even when the work from home mandate went into effect. I found that if I wanted to maintain my fitness goals, I had to adjust my schedule. I started to workout first thing in the morning, and I really loved it. I now find evening workouts more difficult (never thought I would say that). If it really feels too difficult to wake up early, I will work out in the evening instead. However, there have been occasions where I miss a morning workout and an evening as well because of work, so I try my hardest not to miss a workout in the morning if I can help it.

Change the Type of Exercises According to Your Goals

As I mentioned, I have always been doing cardio exercises and probably will continue based on its benefits. However, there came a point in time where I realized that based on my goals I had to change the type of exercises I was doing. For years, I was against any form of strength training; I found it monotonous, and I did not want to look like a man. Since I reached my goal weight and size, I have loose skin and have lost muscle mass. One of the sure ways to help is strength training, much to my detriment. But, since I have a certain goal I want to achieve, I must do these exercises even if I don't like them.

Know Your Numbers

Another important part of living right is taking control of your health and visiting your doctor. It is important to know the current status of your heath. Do not wait until something is wrong before you decide to see a doctor. In a worst-case scenario, your health has already deteriorated. If you *feel* fine, that does not mean you are. For a long time, my blood pressure was high and I never knew it; I felt fine; therefore, I thought I was fine. What was worse is, even when I was first told my blood pressure readings were of concern, I blew it off—big mistake. Please do not do that. I did not even change any of my habits; I ignored the doctor's concerns because of my age, and I felt at the time I had more important things to worry about. Going to the doctor should not only be when something is wrong but as a routine annual wellness visit, or more, depending on the state of your health. For some, I know going to a doctor is a burden, a waste of time, and an expensive venture. Regardless, prevention is always a safer and cheaper alternative than needing to afford a cure.

If cost is a major reason preventing you from visiting a doctor, please do not use that as an excuse. There are a number of places that offer free services to check your blood pressure and cholesterol, especially in the United States where the pharmacies provide some of these services for free. While in Jamaica, there are health fairs that offer these services for free as well; it is a matter of checking newspapers, television, radio, or social media outlets for the available dates. If that is your only choice, I implore you to take advantage of these opportunities because your health depends on it.

The important numbers to know are:

- Blood Sugar
- Blood Pressure
- Blood Cholesterol
- Body Weight

Knowing these numbers is a great start in helping you figure out the state of your health. Now if your numbers are normal, fabulous, keep doing whatever you are doing to maintain it. For those who need improvement or are required to take medication, do not get too discouraged. You are now aware of the problem and are on the road to improving your health. Changing your habits is very important, but you must follow the doctor's orders.

Listen to Your Doctor and Take Your Medication

I have heard a number of success stories of persons who have stopped taking their medication or reversed their health condition completely by changing their habits. But, you must do this along with your doctor's supervision and guidance. Whatever prescription(s) you were given is necessary to help your body function properly until you are able to make consistent healthy eating and exercise habits that will improve your body naturally. Refusing or stopping the medication without your doctor's approval may be harmful. Also, just because you do not *feel* sick does not mean you should stop taking your medication either. In order for you to get better, you must take your medication in conjunction with maintaining a healthy lifestyle. You can work on weaning yourself off the medication whenever your doctor sees improvement. I fought very hard to reduce my medication; I constantly pleaded with my doctor at every visit to get me off the medication. It took a long time to start lowering my dosage, but I worked hard at it. I took my pills consistently and regularly, and I was mindful of what I ate, and included exercise. Getting off medication is easier for some; for others, it is not, but it is definitely possible. In order to achieve this, you must have a plan in place.

Set a Goal and Make it SMART

Whatever goals you have in mind about your health, ensure they fall under the SMART criteria:

S- Specific
M- Measurable
A- Achievable
R- Realistic
T- Time-based

Specific	What exactly do you want to achieve?
	Example: To lose 10 pounds.
Measurable	How will you know you have achieved your goal?
	Example: The number on the scale decreases, clothes are more comfortable.
Action Oriented	Is it achievable?
	Example: Engage in physical activity five times a week, change eating habits.
Realistic	Is it realistic?
	Example: Weigh once every four weeks. Keep a daily food journal
Time	What is your deadline?
	Example: three months

The above table is an example of SMART goals. You can apply this strategy to any goal you want to achieve. If you do not achieve your goals within your time frame, ensure that you make adjustments, see what areas you need to improve on, and keep going. Just because it does not happen within your allotted time frame does not mean you should give up. It may just mean working harder and finding alternative methods until you accomplish your goal.

Chapter 9 Quotes:

- ❖ "I always believed if you take care of your body it will take care of you." —Ted Lindsay
- ❖ "Take care of your body. It's the only place you have to live." —Anonymous
- ❖ "EXERCISE to be fit not skinny. EAT to nourish your body and always IGNORE the haters, doubters and unhealthy examples that were once feeding you. YOU are worth more than you realize." —Anonymous

Chapter 10

Maintaining a Healthy Lifestyle

L osing weight is hard but maintaining it is just as difficult. Having lost over 100 pounds, my fear of regaining the weight and dealing with all the health issues I went through a few years ago will always remain in the back of my mind. I do not want to ever go through that again. However, according to research, "80% of people who successfully lose at least 10% of their body weight will gradually regain it to end up as large or even larger than they were before they went on a diet" (Goodman, 2016). Who or what should be blamed for this, you may ask? Our food intake and metabolism. Our bodies are fighting against the maintenance of the weight we lost (Goodman, 2016). If I think back to all the diets I have tried, this makes sense. Think about it, diets require us to be in a caloric deficit; the minute we go off the diet and begin consuming the foods we denied previously, we inevitably regain the weight lost and maybe even more.

For years, I went on various crash diets, some lasting longer than others. Eventually, what I thought was the magic weight loss formula eventually started being impossible to sustain long term. It was in those moments I felt worthless and could not understand why weight loss seemed like this impossible goal that I would never be able to achieve. Well, long term weight loss is possible. As of March 2021, I am proud to say that I have been maintaining my weight loss for over nine years. In these nine years, I regained at most between 5-15 pounds. That is not bad. The reason my weight loss has been so successful this time around comes down to habits. A lot of the habits I have done in the past, I have limited and or completely eliminated.

Please keep in mind that my previous diet consisted mainly of highly processed foods that were high in fats, sodium and sugars, with very limited intake of fruits and vegetables. My habits today are completely different. I still consume full-fat ice cream and cake but in moderation. I have also managed to be consistent with exercising between 4-5 days weekly. I may have gained some weight, but my focus has been on ensuring that my blood pressure remains under control.

Since I was officially diagnosed with high blood pressure, I had to try multiple medications that worked for me before settling on three high-dose medication combinations. The medications helped; my blood pressure was consistently under control whenever I did my regular check-up. I ensured I took my medication as prescribed, limited my sodium intake, and exercised. Within a few years, I have come down to two medications at the lowest dosage available.

Motivation May Deteriorate but Remain Consistent

At the beginning of my journey, I was extremely motivated and determined to reclaim my health and ensure that my long-term goals of being a certain weight, size, and being off medication completely would come to fruition. As I began marking my goals off the checklist, I noticed that at some point I started slacking off. Now, I was comfortable with my weight and my overall health. My new habits were now second nature, and I focused on other things, whether it was traveling, new jobs, love interests or getting my degree.

I never lost motivation but my focus shifted as various things competed for my attention as my life changed. This is normal; the habits I learned along the way are what kept my health in check.

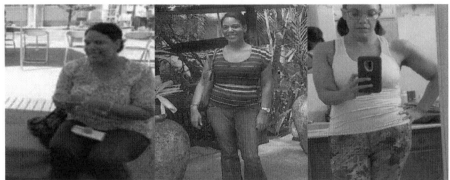

Starting weight:	Goal Weight:	Maintenance weight:
200+ pounds	147 pounds	156 pounds

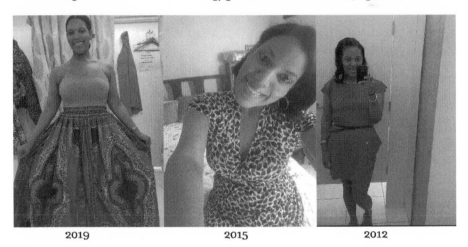

| 2019 | 2015 | 2012 |

Chapter 10 Quotes:

- ❖ "Discipline is the bridge between goals and accomplishment." —Jim Rohn
- ❖ "Motivation may get you started but it takes discipline to keep you going." —John Maxwell
- ❖ "Self-discipline is about controlling your desires and impulses while staying focused on what needs to get done to achieve your goals." —Adam Sicinski

Chapter 11

COVID-19 Pandemic Weight Gain: Causes and Tips to Lose It

As I mentioned in the previous chapter, I have managed to maintain my weight loss for a little over nine years. Throughout those nine years, I dealt with the daily struggles of life and major life changes such as moving to different countries, starting and completing a graduate degree, starting and losing jobs, and romantic relationships. However, never in my wildest dreams would I ever think of adding a pandemic to that list.

When I first heard about the Novel Coronavirus, I literally thought it would be something that would blow over in a matter of months, and everything would be back to normal. It is more than a year later, and many countries are still dealing with a high number of cases and death rates. Along with that, in order to reduce the spread of the virus, countries have implemented restrictions that have influenced how we travel and exist under these new conditions.

In April 2020, in Jamaica, we closed our borders, restaurants, beaches, and non-essential businesses, and the government implemented the work from home orders. As an essential worker, I still had to go to work as cases started being reported in Kingston. It did not feel real until cases were being reported in my office and eventually in persons I interacted with occasionally. I was terrified every day as my exposure increased once I left home. As the situation became more dire I eventually received approval to work from home.

Despite the fact that I was now home, the work had to continue as my responsibilities involved dealing with risk communication aspects of the pandemic. The stress was high, and certain healthy habits went right down the drain. What made matters worse is, I had stopped working out months before. As soon as I decided to begin working out again, all gyms were closed. The desire to workout was gone. The thought of exercising at home never entered my mind. After months of eating and no exercise routine, I decided I had enough. I did not want to allow this situation to undo all my hard work. I knew after months of baking and trying new recipes, I gained some weight. I was officially a member of the *"Quarantine 19"* club.

Since you got this far in my book, you are fully aware of the *"Freshman 15."* Now, there is a new expression, *"Quarantine 19,"* referring to weight gained during the COVID-19 pandemic. According to a poll of 1,000 WebMD readers, approximately half of the women and about one-quarter of the men indicated they gained weight "due to COVID restrictions" (MUHealth, 2020)). These results are not surprising.

I am sure if we took a poll in Jamaica, many persons would say the same thing. Since March 2020, all our routines have been disrupted, leading to an increase in stress, and it is still unclear when or if things will ever return to normal. In the meantime, it is important to understand what got us to put on the weight and implement some tips to reverse it.

Causes of Weight Gain

During this pandemic, the three main culprits of weight gain are stress/emotional eating, being physically inactive, and our mental health (O'Connor, 2020). These main causes are interlinked and affect us all differently.

Sedentary Lifestyle

Many countries had to close facilities (gyms, parks, schools) that promote physical activity in order to minimize the spread of COVID. These closures, though for the benefit of our health, have ironically been detrimental to our health. Studies are now showing that the average person is spending more time on social media, watching television, and sitting. In addition to inactivity, persons are not only eating more; they are eating foods that are fattier and less healthy (O'Connor, 2020).

Stress/Emotional Eating

Whenever I am sad or upset, I always find myself resorting to food, specifically ice cream. Does this sound familiar? This is emotional eating. This is considered a common practice and is done during stressful circumstances, from work stress to relationship problems and health issues. Emotional eating affects both men and women; however, it is more common in women (Marcin, 2018). So, what is the reason we resort to food? According to Ashley Marcin, author of, *"Emotional Eating: What You Should know,"* "Food is believed to be a way to fill that void and create a false feeling of 'fullness' or 'temporary wholeness'" (Marcin, 2018). Additional reasons are:

- Withdrawing from social support in times of emotional need.

- Not engaging in activities that relieve stress or sadness.
- Not understanding the difference between physical and emotional hunger.
- Using negative self-talk that is related to bingeing episodes.
- Changing cortisol levels in response to stress, which leads to cravings. (Marcin, 2018).

Mental Health

Technology has increased our social interaction more than ever in the last few years. I am able to chat with my friends and family with the press of a button. COVID has forced us to rely on technology now more than ever to communicate with our loved ones and to protect them and ourselves. This has forced us to see how valuable human contact and physical interactions are for our emotional well-being. I never thought one day simple gestures of a handshake or a hug could potentially put your health at risk. Again, even though we must limit physical interactions to slow the spread of this deadly disease, it is at a cost to our mental well-being.

Over the past year, I have seen the different ways the infection and prevention protocols have affected not only my eating habits but my mental well-being, such as reminding myself to carry adequate supplies of hand sanitizers and wipes every time I go outside, washing my hands multiple times daily after touching high touch surfaces, and the mental exercise of worrying if I washed my hands and sanitized surfaces properly. There are days I get sick and tired of being home in the same room and staring at a computer day after day; I have had enough of it. I miss traveling. I miss the simple things like going to the supermarket or bank without constantly having to remind people to keep their distance and not having to wear a mask. I miss going to movies or hotels without the increased risk of catching COVID. Worse, persons have experienced job loss, business loss, the guilt of exposing their loved ones to this disease and grief from the death of loved ones, and so much more. This pandemic has been trying, and no matter how small or big, we must find ways to cope.

No one has an exact date on when this pandemic will be over. The vaccine has been implemented in many countries and the more persons get vaccinated the quicker those countries will be able to have herd immunity and get back to some version of normalcy. However, until then, we should make some attempt at applying some tips and strategies to help during this time.

Tips to Losing the Quarantine Weight

Create a Daily Routine

Whether you are still working from home or back at your workplace, you must create a routine to give your day some structure. Having a daily routine will make your life easier and more efficient. Your routine should be based on the goals you would like to achieve. Therefore, if you want to lose weight, plan your days so that they will be conducive towards that goal. Realistically speaking, things can go wrong that will force you to alter your plans. For example, unexpected meetings can cause you to skip your workout or miss lunch or you can forget your lunch because you were rushing to leave home, so you have to resort to takeout. You could also be forced to eat what is at home because supermarkets closed early due to a curfew order issued to curtail the pandemic. Whatever the problem is, simply adjust the rest of the day and do your best.

Think about What You are Eating

During the lockdown, you may have found yourself snacking and generally eating more than usual while not necessarily keeping track of the quantity and frequency of your snacking. It is important to start tracking your foods. You can start keeping a food diary and monitor all the foods you have been eating. Write down everything, even when you take the sample at the supermarket or just lick the spoon with cake batter. By doing this, you have a visual representation of what changes you need to make. Then you can use this information to create a plan. Implement SMART goal and ask yourself these questions:

What is my goal? (e.g., to lose 10 pounds)

_____

_____

_____

_____

What food(s) do I need to remove to help achieve my goal?

_____

_____

_____

_____

What foods can I eat instead to replace the removed item? (e.g., sweetened fruit-filled yogurt/plain unsweetened Greek yogurt)

_____

_____

_____

_____

Do I plan to exercise? If so, how often?

_____

_____

_____

_____

Will I do meal prep? What is the best day for me to meal prep?

_____

_____

_____

_____

What factors can I think of that will negatively affect me from reaching my goals?

_____

_____

_____

_____

Exercise (Schedule Regular Exercise)

We have heard it time and time again to exercise and do it daily. A lot of the weight gain comes not only from eating too much but also from not burning off the excess calories. Now let me be real and honest, you can certainly lose weight without exercise. Science has proven it, and there are several examples of persons who have been successful. However, I strongly recommend that you engage in some form of physical activity, even if it means walking around in circles in your own house. Exercise does not have to be complicated or difficult, it can be as simple as gardening or walking up a flight of stairs. Physical activity not only helps us to lose weight, it also impacts our overall health, which is crucial in these times. The benefits of exercise, according to Ashley Marcin, are:

- It can make you feel happier (exercise improves your mood and decreases feelings of depression, anxiety, and stress)
- It aids in building strong muscles and bones
- Increased energy levels
- Reduced risk of chronic diseases
- It helps skin health
- It helps brain health and memory
- It helps with relaxation and sleep quality
- Reduce pain
- Promotes a better sex life (Marcin, 2018)

These benefits all sound so wonderful and are critical to our overall health. As mentioned, you do not need to do anything that is physically strenuous and difficult. It can be as simple as walking, but if you are looking for something with a challenge, I suggest you try activities that you will enjoy. Do not do activities that you hate because you are less likely to continue doing it. Do activities that make you excited to go back again and again.

Sleep

Earlier, I mentioned the importance of exercising and watching your eating habits. Well, getting a good night's sleep is just as important. Here are ten reasons how sleep affects our overall health.

1. **"Poor sleep is linked to higher body weight.**
   a. The effects of sleep on weight gain are multi-factorial, for example, hormones and motivation to

exercise. Therefore, if you want to lose weight, quality sleep is important.

2. **Good sleepers tend to eat fewer calories.**
    a. Poor quality sleep affects the hormones that regulate appetite. Persons who get satisfactory sleep tend to eat fewer calories compared to those who do not.

3. **Good sleep can improve concentration and productivity.**
    a. Good sleep can improve problem-solving skills and boost memory.

4. **Good sleep can maximize athletic performance.**
    a. Longer sleep has been shown to improve many facets of athletic and physical performance.

5. **Poor sleepers have a greater risk of heart disease and stroke.**
    a. Sleeping less than seven or eight hours is associated with an increased risk of heart disease and stroke.

6. **Sleep affects glucose metabolism and type 2 diabetes risk.**
    a. Poor sleeping habits are strongly related to adverse effects on blood sugar levels.

7. **Poor sleep is associated with depression.**
    a. Especially those with a sleep disorder.

8. **Sleep improves your immune function.**
    a. Sleep improves your immune function and helps to fight the common cold.

9. **Poor sleep is linked to increased inflammation.**
    a. Sleep affects your body's inflammatory responses and is linked to inflammatory bowel disease and can increase your risk of the disease reoccurring.

10. **Sleep affects emotions and social interactions.**
    a. Poor quality sleep affects social skills and the ability to recognize emotional expressions. (Leech, 2020)

Now that you know the multiple health risks associated with poor quality sleep. Here are eight tips to help get good quality sleep as stated by Harvard Health:

- **Exercise** - Can be as simple as a walk and exercising in the morning. Studies have shown that exercising in the morning makes it easier to fall asleep in comparison to exercising closer to bedtime.

- **Reserve bedtime for sleep and sex** – So, no phone calls, checking or responding to emails, and watching television.

- **Start a sleep ritual** - Have a set time to go to bed. Do things that signal it is time to go to bed—for example, having a relaxing bath and drinking chamomile tea or warm milk.

- **Avoid overeating** - Avoid eating a large meal before bed. If you are hungry, eat a light snack like an apple or crackers.

- **Stay away from alcohol and caffeine** - These things are stimulants and disrupt your sleep.

- **De-stress** - Many of us have stressful events and situations going on throughout the day; it is important to try and put those things away before bedtime. Learn relaxation techniques or deep breathing exercises to help promote good sleep.

- **Get checked** - If you are ever experiencing symptoms of burning pain in the stomach, chest, or throat, movement in the legs, or even snoring, there could be some serious health conditions going on, especially if they are keeping you awake at night. If so, please see a doctor for a checkup. (Harvard Health, 2012).

Manage Stress

More stress

=

More cortisol

=

Higher appetite for junk food

=

More belly fat

(Breeze, 2016)

When we are stressed, our body releases the stress hormone, cortisol. This hormone increases your insulin levels, then "your blood sugar drops, and you crave sugary fatty foods" (Breeze, 2016). This explains why we resort to comfort food like cookies and macaroni and cheese instead of fruits or vegetables. According to experts, "eating can be a source of solace and can lower stress. This happens in part because the body releases chemicals in response to food that might have a direct calming effect" (Breeze, 2016). Unfortunately, too much weight can lead to a number of health issues such as high blood pressure, diabetes, heart disease, and stroke. Therefore, it is important to deal with stress. Here are some techniques or strategies to help you cope:

Positive Self-Talk

We all say things to ourselves, whether we want to admit it or not. If we think about it, a lot of it may be more negative than we realize. It is this negative self-talk that can increase stress. Instead, we should do the reverse. Try this; make a list of five negative things you usually say to yourself and then write down the positive one for it. For example,

Negative Statements	Positive Statements
"I can't do this"	I can do this
	I will do the best I can
	I have got this
"This is too hard"	This is solvable
	I can find solutions to this problem (AHA, 2014).

Practice Stress Techniques

Think of different actions that you can use to help solve whatever is making you feel stressed. You may need to apply different techniques for different situations such as:

- Exercise
- Meditation
- Breaking down problems into small parts. Doing each thing one piece at a time.
- Listening to music

- Take breaks (AHA, 2014)

Engage in Activities that You Enjoy

One of the best ways to de-stress is doing things that you enjoy and make you happy, for example:

- Drawing, painting, playing an instrument
- Listening to music
- Reading a book
- Sports
- Picking up a hobby
- Taking a bath
- Getting fresh air (walking outside for ten minutes)

(AHA, 2014)

If any of these suggested techniques do not work for you, I implore you to talk to a family member, friend, or a trained professional. Please seek help; you are not alone no matter what you are going through.

Chapter 11 Quotes:

- ❖ "Every new day is another chance to change your life." — Anonymous
- ❖ "You didn't gain all your weight in one day; you won't lose it in one day. Be patient with yourself." —Jenna Wolfe
- ❖ "21/90 Rule: It takes 21 days to create a habit, 90 days to create a lifestyle." —Anonymous

Chapter 12

Inspire U

It has been nine years since I decided to make the change to live a healthy lifestyle, and I am amazed at what I have accomplished. Losing over 100 pounds is a huge achievement, and I am so unbelievably proud of myself. This was not just for my physical appearance, but it was a shedding of my insecurities and all the negative things I used to believe and think about myself. It was an unveiling of the person that was meant to be under all that weight. It has also been a journey of unlearning old habits and replacing them with new ones. Even though I have been on this journey for a while, I am still learning.

As you have just read, my journey has been slow but successful and filled with obstacles and battles I had to overcome. What I want you to take away from all of this is:

1. *Figure out your why.* Whatever your *why* is, it should be the motivating reason for you to start your journey.

2. *Everyone's journey is different*. Therefore, do not compare your progress. I know it is easier said than done, but remember our bodies are different, and what affects me may not be an issue for someone else. I may work out six days per week and limit certain foods for weeks and still not show

any improvement. While someone else who did the exact thing not only lost weight but went down a full-dress size. You may reach your goal sooner than anticipated, and that would be amazing; or like me, you may need more time, and that is okay. It is your journey.

3. *Make small changes*. You have a goal but it just seems impossible and there are too many things you need to do. Relax, this process should not make you feel so overwhelmed that you want to quit before you even start. Make small changes one step at a time and slowly add new goals along the way.

4. *Slow progress is progress.* This is not a race; this is a journey, and it will take some time. Therefore, please do not rely on the scale alone. Look at how your clothes feel. Do you notice that you are drinking more water than you did before, or are you able to walk ten minutes more than you did the previous week or month? Are you noticing that you have more energy than you did a couple of weeks ago? Are you eating more fruits and vegetables than you ever have in your life? Have your test results improved? This journey is not just about your weight loss but improvements in your overall health and wellness.

5. *Do what is best for you.* As you know by now, I am an advocate for living a healthy lifestyle, and it is when you change your habits that you are more likely to sustain long-term results. However, I believe whatever journey you choose to take is ultimately up to you. Try some of the strategies and apply it and see if it works.

6. ***Do not give up.*** Let us say you gained weight or hit a plateau and even remained there for weeks. You are tempted to throw in the proverbial towel; do not. Adjust and keep trying. You will make mistakes along the way, and that is life. Learn from them and try again.

7. ***Be consistent.*** To see results, you must be consistent. Over time, motivation will slowly disappear, but you must remind yourself of your *why* at some point. Discipline will help to keep you on your journey.

8. ***Surround yourself with people who will support you and your journey.*** As you make changes for the better, you might encounter friends or even family members who may not be supportive. It may be through jokes, snide remarks, criticisms or simply an unwillingness to adapt to the changes. That is okay. Remember, this is about you and your journey. Share with your immediate family members and close friends why you are doing this and that you may need their support. Be open and honest as well; if that does not work, use whatever negative comments they may say as motivation. Through this new journey, I guarantee you will find persons with the same goals who will encourage and provide you with the support you need.

I shared my story with you all because I honestly never thought I would ever lose weight. As you have read, I tried many diets over time and failed repeatedly. Many of those diets did not work because I was focused on the wrong things. This time I focused on my health and made the necessary changes to my habits; I can safely say it has worked. I have kept off a majority of the weight for over nine years and have seen improvement in my blood pressure and other key areas. I believe this way of life will work for you with patience and consistency. You can use the next set of pages as a guide to help motivate and encourage you to start your journey to living a healthy lifestyle.

Happy healthy makeover!

Chapter 12 Quotes:

* ❖ "Start with changing unhealthy habits to healthy ones and make them your favorites." —Sahara Sanders
* ❖ "Start where you are. Use what you have. Do what you can." —Arthur Ashe
* ❖ "Stop doubting yourself and start taking action. I don't care how small that first step may seem. There comes a time when you just need to dive right in." —Anonymous
* ❖ "Only I can change my life, no one can do it for me." — Anonymous

How to Start Your Own Healthy Makeover

Congratulations! You finished reading about my health journey and the steps I took to get my health back on track and lose weight. I hope everything you have read has inspired and motivated you to adopt new, healthier habits. The rest of this chapter will provide you with the steps and strategies to begin your own healthy makeover.

Before you begin, according to the research conducted by the National Institute of Diabetes and Digestive and Kidney Diseases, you must first identify and recognize the four stages of changing your behavior (N.I.D.D.K.D., n.d.). The Stages of Change Model or Transtheoretical Model was developed in the late 1970s and "operates on the assumption that people do not change behaviors quickly and decisively. Rather, change in behavior, especially habitual behavior, occurs continuously through a cyclical process" (LaMorte, 2019). Knowing the different stages will determine the type of actions that you are willing to take in order to achieve your goal(s). The five stages of behavior change are:

- Contemplation
- Preparation
- Action

- Maintenance
- Relapse

Contemplation (I am thinking about it)

This is the first stage. In the contemplation stage, it means you are thinking about making some changes and becoming motivated to start (N.I.D.D.K.D., n.d.). If you are at this stage, then you may:

- Be considering a change but not ready yet.
- Believe your overall health will improve if you develop new habits.
- Be unsure of how you will overcome obstacles which is what is keeping you from starting (N.I.D.D.K.D., n.d.).

If you are at this stage, making any kind of change is hard especially if it is something you have never done before.

Action Steps to Take:

Make a benefits and challenge or pros and cons list of changing your habits.

Goal: _____

Benefits/Pros	Challenges/Cons

Now look at the list and think about how you can overcome those challenges. The next stage will help you do that.

Preparation (My mind is made up, and I am ready to take action)

This is the second stage. At this stage, you are already making plans and have thought of specific ideas on what will work for you (N.I.D.D.K.D., n.d.). If you are at this stage, then you may:

- Have made the decisions to change and are ready to take action.
- Have some specific goals you would like to achieve.
- Be getting ready to put your plan into action (N.I.D.D.K.D., n.d.).

In the preparation stage, you created a list of benefits and challenges of achieving your goal.

Action Steps to Take:

Now look at this list and put it into action for those challenges or obstacles. Write down the solution to them.

Challenges/Obstacles	Solution

Now that you have written down some of the foreseeable challenges, you should feel a lot more comfortable and ready to take action. Now it is time to make a plan.

Action Steps to Take:

- Do some research about your goal. For example, if your goal is to eat healthier, visit websites about healthy eating or physical activity.
- Make lists of healthy foods that you like and should get more of that are within your budget.
- Make a list of foods you need to reduce or eliminate from your diet and their alternatives.
- Make a list of physical activities that you would enjoy and the fitness centers you want to use or home workout videos (N.I.D.D.K.D., n.d.).

Now you should be ready to set your goal and put it into action. Remember to start small and achieve one goal at a time.

Action Steps to Take:

Complete the following:

1. Healthy Makeover Starter Questionnaire
2. My Healthy Makeover SMART Action Plan

Action (I have started making changes)

In the third stage, you will now act on the plan you made and are ready to achieve your goal. If you are at this stage, then you:

- Have made some behavior changes within 3-6 months.
- Are getting used to or adjusted those behavior changes.
- Have overcome the challenges or obstacles (N.I.D.D.K.D., n.d.).

Maintenance (I have new routines)

This is the fourth stage. Here you have gotten used to the changes and have been keeping it up for six months or more. If you are at this stage, then you:

- Have made changes that are now a part of your normal routine.
- Have found creative and innovative ways to stick to your routine.
- Have experienced setbacks and were able to get past them and make progress.

Please note that this phase can last for years (N.I.D.D.K.D., n.d.).

Relapse

The fifth and final stage is the relapse stage. Relapses or setbacks are common and to be expected (Cherry, 2020). When this happens, you are going to feel frustrated, disappointed, and even "feel like a failure." The best way to overcome these feelings is to focus on why this setback happened and what triggered it (Cherry, 2020). Start again and begin evaluating the preparation, action, and maintenance stages of the behavior change model. Go through your action plan and your goals and make adjustments where necessary. Keep making modifications to your plans as much as you need to until you figure out what works. Remember, health is a journey and not a destination. Be patient with yourself and the process, and keep going no matter how long it takes.

Now Consider the Following:

After reading the above stages, can you identify your current stage of change? Once you have identified your stage within the behavior change model, you can now take the necessary affiliated action-orientated and SMART steps to achieve your goals. Please be aware that in order to be truly successful, I recommend following all action steps within each phase of the behavior change model.

Remember, this book can be used as a guide to help you achieve your goals. So, go through it slowly, and I hope this will help you in your health journey. Thank you.

My Healthy Makeover Starter Questionnaire

When was your last wellness or doctor's appointment? (If it was over a year ago, go schedule a visit whether virtually or face to face)

_____Write the date

Did you get a blood test done? □ Yes □ No (If no, see if the doctor needs to schedule one)

Were the results good or bad?

Did your doctor ask you to make any lifestyle changes? □ Yes □ No

(If yes, answer the next question. Even if your answer is no, answer anyway. We all need to make changes no matter how small.)

What changes do you need to make? (List top 3 changes)

1)_____

2)_____

3)_____

List your top 3 health goals (e.g., eat more fruits and vegetables, drink more water, etc.)

1)_____

2) _____

3) _____

Now that you are aware of your current health status and you identified what changes you need to make and the goals you want to achieve, the next step is to create a plan. An action plan will outline the necessary steps to achieve your goal and reach your target within an assigned time frame. The first thing is, you must make your goals SMART like I discussed earlier.

Helpful Tips

1. Concentrate on one goal at a time. Doing too much may be overwhelming and may cause you to fail.
2. Choose a goal that you feel you are ready to accomplish.
3. Start small. The goal should be challenging but attainable.
4. Get support. Ask a friend to be your accountability partner or find a support group.
5. Refer to your action plan daily to keep you on track and log your progress. Doing this will keep you motivated.
6. Revaluate your progress often. If something is working, continue it, and if something is not, make the necessary changes.
7. Set new goals every three months.

My Healthy Makeover SMART Action Plan

Write down one area you want to improve/change:

BE SPECIFIC (*what do you want* *to achieve*)	I will_____
MEASURABLE (*how will you* *track your* *progress*)	I will_____
ACTION- **ORIENTED** (*identify an action* *that will help you* *reach your goal*)	I will_____
REALISTIC (*set a goal that is* *realistic*)	I will_____
TIME (*set a start and* *end date*)	_____

My Healthy Makeover SMART Action Plan

Write down one area you want to improve/change:

BE SPECIFIC (*what do you want* *to achieve*)	I will_____
MEASURABLE (*how will you* *track your* *progress*)	I will_____
ACTION- **ORIENTED** (*identify an action* *that will help you* *reach your goal*)	I will_____
REALISTIC (*set a goal that is* *realistic*)	I will_____
TIME (*set a start and* *end date*)	_____

My Healthy Makeover SMART Action Plan

Write down one area you want to improve/change:

BE SPECIFIC *(what do you want to achieve)*	I will_____
MEASURABLE *(how will you track your progress)*	I will_____
ACTION-ORIENTED *(identify an action that will help you reach your goal)*	I will_____
REALISTIC *(set a goal that is realistic)*	I will_____
TIME *(set a start and end date)*	_____

Recipes

No Fuss Oatmeal

½ cup old fashion oats

½ cup water

½ tsp. cinnamon

1 banana

Optional Topping Items:

½ tsp. chopped almonds

½ tsp. chopped walnuts

½ tsp. pumpkin seeds

¼ cup of chopped apples

Instructions:

Cook oatmeal according to directions. Top with banana, cinnamon, or optional toppings.

Kale Me Up Green Smoothie

2 cups of kale (stems removed)

1 cup of spinach

½ cup of pineapple

1 cup water or coconut water

Optional Items:

1 tsp. Chlorella

1 banana or ¼ cup mango (if you desire extra sweetness)

Instructions:
Remove stems from kale and wash along with spinach in cold water before use. Place all ingredients in a high-powered blender and blend until smooth.

Vegan Fettuccine Alfredo
Alfredo Sauce:
¼ white onion
2 medium white potatoes (can substitute with ½ cup cauliflower)
½ cup raw cashews
3 cloves of garlic
½ of juice from lemon
1 cup of water

Optional:
½ tsp salt and black pepper to taste

Enjoy with:
Whole-wheat pasta
Zucchini or Squash noodles

Add ons:
½ cup spinach
½ cup broccoli
¼ white or red onions
¼ green, red or yellow peppers

Instructions:
Boil water with onion and potatoes and cook until potatoes are tender.

While potatoes are cooking, add cashews, lemon juice, and garlic to a blender and set aside.

Once potatoes and onions are cooked, add to blender. Add ½ cup of water used to cook potatoes, salt, and pepper and blend in a *NutriBullet* or high-powered blender. Blend until smooth. Add more of the water based on desired thickness.

Add sauce to cooked pasta or zucchini or squash noodles and add extra veggies to make it more filling and nutritious.

Coconut Curry Chickpeas
1 can of low sodium chickpeas
1 white onion
1 green pepper
3 cloves of garlic
2 stalks of scallion
1 tbsp. coconut oil
¼ cup of coconut milk
2 tbsp. of curry powder
¼ tsp. onion powder
¼ tsp. black pepper
¼ tsp. Mrs. Dash seasoning

Optional Add Ins:
¼ cup roasted cashews

¼ cup mixed vegetables (frozen or canned)
1 small white potato cubed

Instructions:

Drain the can of chickpeas and set aside—place oil in a frying pan on medium-low heat. Add curry powder to hot oil and stir. Carefully add a couple of teaspoons of hot water to curry and stir until curry powder dissolves. Add coconut milk, stir, and simmer for 10 minutes. Add Mrs. Dash, onion, green pepper, scallion, black pepper, onion powder, and garlic. Stir and cook for 10 minutes. Add chickpeas or optional cashews and potatoes* and simmer for another 10 minutes. Serve over brown/white rice or cauliflower rice, or quinoa with steamed veggies.

*If adding potatoes, you can cook separately and add them last or cook it with curry.

About the Author

Stacy Wright was born and raised in Jamaica. For over twenty-eight years, she was significantly overweight, tried various fad diets, failed, and always regained the weight. Out of concern for her own health and the need for more health education in Jamaica, Stacy obtained her Master's in Public Health and became a Certified Health Education Specialist. Her goal is to provide others with the knowledge and skills to gain control over their health and to recognize that becoming healthy is a life-long journey. She considers herself the adventurous type and loves traveling. She has lived in the United States and Japan and has traveled throughout North America, Central America, Asia, and the Caribbean.

References

3 Tips to Manage Stress. (n.d.). Www.Heart.Org. Retrieved March 14, 2021, from https://www.heart.org/en/healthy-living/healthy-lifestyle/stress-management/3-tips-to-manage-stress

Ahn, K. (2015, August 13). *How To: Eat Better by Making Healthy Food More Visible*. WonderHowTo. https://food-hacks.wonderhowto.com/how-to/eat-better-by-making-healthy-food-more-visible-0156446/

American Heart Association Recommendations for Physical Activity in Adults and Kids. (n.d.). Www.Heart.Org. Retrieved June 28, 2021, from https://www.heart.org/en/healthy-living/fitness/fitness-basics/aha-recs-for-physical-activity-in-adults

BeLue, R., Francis, L. A., & Colaco, B. (2009). Mental Health Problems and Overweight in a Nationally Representative Sample of Adolescents: Effects of Race and Ethnicity. *PEDIATRICS*, *123*(2), 697–702. https://doi.org/10.1542/peds.2008-0687

Biro, F. M., & Wien, M. (2010). Childhood obesity and adult morbidities. *The American Journal of Clinical Nutrition*, *91*(5), 1499S-1505S. https://doi.org/10.3945/ajcn.2010.28701b

Breeze, J. (2016, February 9). *Can Stress Cause Weight Gain?* WebMD. https://www.webmd.com/diet/features/stress-weight-gain#1

Changing Your Habits for Better Health. (n.d.). National Institute of Diabetes and Digestive and Kidney Diseases. Retrieved April

21, 2021, from https://www.niddk.nih.gov/health-information/diet-nutrition/changing-habits-better-health

Cherry, K. (2020, November 9). *The 6 Stages of Behavior Change.* Verywell Mind. https://www.verywellmind.com/the-stages-of-change-2794868

Chiang, J. (2015, August 1). *Hypertension and Diabetic Kidney Disease in Children and Adolescents.* Diabetes Spectrum. https://spectrum.diabetesjournals.org/content/28/3/220

Cooper, B. (2013, December 5). *The Science of Self-Control: 6 Ways to Improve Your Willpower Today.* Buffer. https://buffer.com/resources/willpower-and-the-brain-why-its-so-hard-to-avoid-temptation/

Defining Adult Overweight and Obesity. (2021, June 7). Centers for Disease Control and Prevention. https://www.cdc.gov/obesity/adult/defining.html

Deliens, T., Clarys, P., de Bourdeaudhuij, I., & Deforche, B. (2014). Determinants of eating behaviour in university students: a qualitative study using focus group discussions. *BMC Public Health, 14*(1). https://doi.org/10.1186/1471-2458-14-53

Dietary Guidelines for Americans, 2020–2025. Executive Summary. (2020). USDA. https://www.dietaryguidelines.gov/resources/2020-2025-dietary-guidelines-online-materials

Duke Medicine. (2013, June 18). *Parenting and home environment influence children's exercise and eating habits.* ScienceDaily. https://www.sciencedaily.com/releases/2013/06/130618113652.htm

Exercise: 7 benefits of regular physical activity. (2019, May 11). Mayo Clinic. https://www.mayoclinic.org/healthy-lifestyle/fitness/in-depth/exercise/art-20048389

Facts About Hypertension | cdc.gov. (2020, September 8). Centers for Disease Control and Prevention. https://www.cdc.gov/bloodpressure/facts.htm

Figueroa, J., Harris, M., Duncan, J., & Tulloch-Reid, M. (2017). Hypertension Control: The Caribbean Needs Intervention Studies to Learn How to Do Better. *West Indian Medical Journal*. Published. https://doi.org/10.7727/wimj.2017.073

Food Labeling: Revision of the Nutrition and Supplement Facts Labels. (2016, May 26). FDA. https://www.regulations.gov/document/FDA-2012-N-1210-0875

Goodman, B. (2016, October 14). *How Your Appetite Can Sabotage Weight Loss*. WebMD. https://www.webmd.com/diet/news/20161014/how-your-appetite-can-sabotage-weight-loss#1

Gunnars, K. B. (2021, June 10). *Daily Intake of Sugar — How Much Sugar Should You Eat Per Day?* Healthline. https://www.healthline.com/nutrition/how-much-sugar-per-day#section3

Harding, G. (2017, October 10). *Why kids want to eat processed foods (& how to change that)*. Well Nourished. https://wellnourished.com.au/why-kids-want-processed-food/

Harvard Health. (2012, July 1). *8 secrets to a good night's sleep*. https://www.health.harvard.edu/sleep/8-secrets-to-a-good-nights-sleep

Harvard Health. (2019, June 24). *Why people become overweight*. https://www.health.harvard.edu/staying-healthy/why-people-become-overweight

High Blood Pressure and African Americans. (n.d.). Www.Heart.Org. Retrieved May 9, 2019, from https://www.heart.org/en/health-topics/high-blood-pressure/why-high-blood-pressure-is-a-silent-killer/high-blood-pressure-and-african-americans

High blood pressure (hypertension) - Symptoms and causes. (2021, January 16). Mayo Clinic. https://www.mayoclinic.org/diseases-conditions/high-blood-pressure/symptoms-causes/syc-20373410

Home | Herbalife Nutrition U.S. (n.d.). Herbalife. Retrieved March 27, 2020, from https://www.herbalife.com/

Jacewicz, N. (2017, May 5). *Why Taste Buds Dull As We Age*. NPR. https://choice.npr.org/index.html?origin=https://www.npr.org/sections/thesalt/2017/05/05/526750174/why-taste-buds-dull-as-we-age

Justus, N. (n.d.). *Why do most diets fail*. Diabetes Councill. https://www.thediabetescouncil.com/why-do-most-diets-fail/

Katella, K. (2020, July 1). *Quarantine 15? What to Do About Weight Gain During the Pandemic*. Yale Medicine. https://www.yalemedicine.org/news/quarantine-15-weight-gain-pandemic

LaMorte, W. W. (2019). *The Transtheoretical Model (Stages of Change)*. Boston University School of Public Health. https://sphweb.bumc.bu.edu/otlt/mph-modules/sb/behavioralchangetheories/behavioralchangetheories6.html

Leech, M. J. S. (2020, February 25). *10 Reasons Why Good Sleep Is Important*. Healthline. https://www.healthline.com/nutrition/10-reasons-why-good-sleep-is-important#10.-Sleep-affects-emotions-and-social-interactions

Live Healthy | MU Health Care. (n.d.). LiveHealthy. Retrieved April 9, 2021, from https://livehealthy.muhealth.org/our-stories/pandemic-weight-gain-its-thing

Marcin, A. (2018, August 29). *Emotional Eating: What You Should Know*. Healthline. https://www.healthline.com/health/emotional-eating

Migala, J. (2018, April 30). *What happens to your brain when you go on a diet*. NBC News. https://www.nbcnews.com/better/health/what-happens-your-brain-when-you-go-diet-ncna802626

Ministry Releases Health and Lifestyle Survey – Jamaica Information Service. (2018, September 6). Jamaica Information Service -

The Voice of Jamaica. https://jis.gov.jm/ministry-releases-health-and-lifestyle-survey/

More than 100 million Americans have high blood pressure, AHA says. (2018, May 1). Www.Heart.Org. https://www.heart.org/en/news/2018/05/01/more-than-100-million-americans-have-high-blood-pressure-aha-says

Muntner, P., Abdalla, M., Correa, A., Griswold, M., Hall, J. E., Jones, D. W., Mensah, G. A., Sims, M., Shimbo, D., Spruill, T. M., Tucker, K. L., & Appel, L. J. (2017). Hypertension in Blacks. *Hypertension, 69*(5), 761–769. https://doi.org/10.1161/hypertensionaha.117.09061

Nania, R. (2017, July 5). *Secret to a long, healthy life? Change your environment.* WTOP. https://wtop.com/health-fitness/2017/07/secret-to-a-long-healthy-life-change-your-environment/

New ACC/AHA High Blood Pressure Guidelines Lower Definition of Hypertension. (2017, November 8). American College of Cardiology. https://www.acc.org/latest-in-cardiology/articles/2017/11/08/11/47/mon-5pm-bp-guideline-aha-2017

New report says obesity on the rise in the Caribbean. (2017, January 19). Jamaica Observer. https://www.jamaicaobserver.com/news/new-report-says-obesity-on-the-rise-in-the-caribbean

Obesity and overweight. (2021, June 9). WHO. https://www.who.int/news-room/fact-sheets/detail/obesity-and-overweight

O'Connor, A. (2020, December 10). *Weight Gain and Stress Eating Are Downside of Pandemic Life.* The New York Times. https://www.nytimes.com/2020/12/04/well/live/pandemic-weight-gain.html

Overweight and Obesity | NHLBI, NIH. (2021, June 23). NIH. https://www.nhlbi.nih.gov/health-topics/overweight-and-obesity

Peeke, P. (2010, April 15). *"Dieting" is Stressful: Ditch the Diet Mentality*. WebMD. https://blogs.webmd.com/from-our-archives/20100415/dieting-is-stressful-ditch-the-diet-mentality

Preidt, R. (2016, December 26). *Wiser, But Fatter, by Graduation*. WebMD. https://www.webmd.com/diet/news/20161226/wiser-but-fatter-by-graduation

Pyper, E., Harrington, D., & Manson, H. (2016). The impact of different types of parental support behaviours on child physical activity, healthy eating, and screen time: a cross-sectional study. *BMC Public Health, 16*(1). https://doi.org/10.1186/s12889-016-3245-0

Semeco, M. A. S. (2017, February 10). *The Top 10 Benefits of Regular Exercise*. Healthline. https://www.healthline.com/nutrition/10-benefits-of-exercise

Sodium sources: Where does all that sodium come from? (n.d.). Www.Heart.Org. Retrieved April 27, 2019, from https://www.heart.org/en/healthy-living/healthy-eating/eat-smart/sodium/sodium-sources

Steakley, L., Goldman, B., & MacCormick, H. (2011, December 29). *The science of willpower*. Scope. https://scopeblog.stanford.edu/2011/12/29/a-conversation-about-the-science-of-willpower/

Strength and Resistance Training Exercise. (n.d.). Www.Heart.Org. Retrieved April 12, 2021, from https://www.heart.org/en/healthy-living/fitness/fitness-basics/strength-and-resistance-training-exercise

Types of exercise | Health Information | Bupa UK. (n.d.). Bupa. Retrieved May 27, 2020, from https://www.bupa.co.uk/health-information/exercise-fitness/types-of-exercise

User, S. (n.d.). *Hypertension - The National Health Fund.* NHF. Retrieved June 26, 2021, from https://www.nhf.org.jm/hypertension

Water and Healthier Drinks. (2021, January 12). Centers for Disease Control and Prevention. https://www.cdc.gov/healthyweight/healthy_eating/water-and-healthier-drinks.html?CDC_AA_refVal=https%3A%2F%2Fwww.cdc.gov%2Fhealthywater%2Fdrinking%2Fnutrition%2Findex.html

Watson, S. (2013, December 10). *The Cabbage Soup Diet.* WebMD. https://www.webmd.com/diet/a-z/cabbage-soup-diet

What are the Symptoms of High Blood Pressure? (n.d.). Www.Heart.Org. Retrieved April 18, 2021, from https://www.heart.org/en/health-topics/high-blood-pressure/why-high-blood-pressure-is-a-silent-killer/what-are-the-symptoms-of-high-blood-pressure

Whitbourne, S. K. (2013, May 23). *Fat Talk and Your Self-Image Talking yourself into feeling fat can be harmful to your mental health.* Psychology Today. https://www.psychologytoday.com/us/blog/fulfillment-any-age/201305/fat-talk-and-your-self-image

Made in the USA
Middletown, DE
23 October 2021